PRAISE FOR ANI'S RAW F

"If you've been putting off plans to trim ... that her plan can help you drop 15 pounc ... While claims like these generally sound impossible and gimmicky, Chef Ani calls on nature's fast foods—raw ingredients. . . .[that] can boost immunity and ... Taste for Life

"*Ani's Raw Food Detox* answers your questions and concerns about a raw diet, and . . . offers an easy, all-raw plan that will help you lose up to 15 pounds in 15 days."—*VegNews*

"The most healthy diet plan I've ever seen! Not only does it detox, nourish, and help you lose pounds, it easily teaches you how to stay that way."—Carol Alt, author of *Eating in the Raw*

"The program embraces what Ani calls nature's fast food, namely raw ingredients straight from the refrigerator or shelf that require very little prep time. From Trail Mix cookies that are loaded with nuts, raisins, and sunflower seeds, to a Spicy Bok Choy Soup, the dishes are exciting and innovative."—*Tucson Citizen*

## PRAISE FOR ANI PHYO

"Phyo . . . is one of the leaders of raw food's latest cycle, thanks to the clever, uncomplicated recipes she develops . . . [her] desserts are universally appealing."—*Food & Wine*

"*Ani's Raw Food Essentials* hits all of the basics—and beyond—in its hefty 300+ pages. Written with the beginner in mind, Phyo's comprehensive content makes it perfect for anyone interested in adding more raw, unprocessed, delicious, and healthy meals to their life . . . Phyo's tone is nothing but positive and supportive, encouraging small steps toward a healthier lifestyle and never demanding a 100-percent raw diet—especially not overnight."—*VegNews*

"If you've ... his is a great starter title."—L

"Ani Phyo is fast becoming the go-to girl for all things raw. This book provides over 250 recipes and tips that prove that you don't have to sacrifice flavour to reap the benefits of a raw food diet. Phyo explains that raw food is more than just a diet—it is a way of life. She teaches readers how eating fresh, organic ingredients can affect the way we look, feel and interact with the earth. If you've been thinking about going raw, this book provides easy transitional recipes and techniques to help you painlessly make the change."
—Healthy Magazine

"*Ani's Raw Food Asia* is more than a collection of recipes; it is a comprehensive guide to raw living, providing tips about non-chemical cleaning, the environment, and attitudes that will ensure a healthier, happier person."—Technorati.com

"Ani Phyo guides readers through the fundamentals of raw food preparation in a simple and user-friendly manner. Phyo has left no stone unturned when it comes to this collection of over 250 recipes."—*VegDaily*

"My wife Jeni and I had the pleasure of taste-testing Ani's delicious, healthy, superfood raw chocolate truffles. Ani's approach is down to earth and uncomplicated, which I like. She makes being raw easy."
—Paul Cook, Sex Pistols

"As someone who has just recently discovered raw food and all its glory, Ani's books and recipes have been both inspiring and exciting. The recipes I've made have been delicious and impressed even my non-raw food friends."—Carrie-Anne Moss, Actress

# ANI'S **RAW FOOD** DETOX

The Easy, Satisfying Plan to Get Lighter,
Tighter, and Sexier . . . in 15 Days or Less

## Ani Phyo

Da Capo
LIFE
LONG

A Member of The Perseus Books Group

*May this book help you to launch your life beyond any limitations and all boundaries. May you enjoy a blissful life with no regrets, that's filled with love, joy, laughter, prosperity, and longevity. Happiness is a reflection of our inner health. Laugh lots, and live long.*

Recipes for Banana Wrap for Moist Silky Skin and Fruit Salad to Feed Your Skin, pages 226–227, from *Ani's Raw Food Desserts* (Da Capo Lifelong Books, 2009)

Additional recipes by: Robert Cheeke, Philip McCluskey, Penni Shelton, Angela Stokes-Monarch, Tonya Zavasta

Designed by Jill Shaffer
Illustrations by Antonio Sanchez
Set in 11-point Chaparral Pro and 9-point Benton Sans by Eclipse Publishing Services

Cataloging-in-Publication data for this book is available from the Library of Congress.

First Da Capo Press edition 2012
Originally published as *Ani's 15-Day Fat Blast: A Kick-Ass Plan to Get Lighter, Tighter, and Sexier...Super Fast*
First paperback edition 2013
ISBN 978-0-7382-1522-8 (hardcover)
ISBN 978-0-7382-1651-5 (paperback)

Published by Da Capo Press
A Member of the Perseus Books Group
www.dacapopress.com

Note: The information in this book is true and complete to the best of our knowledge. This book is intended only as an informative guide for those wishing to know more about health issues. In no way is this book intended to replace, countermand, or conflict with the advice given to you by your own physician. The ultimate decision concerning care should be made between you and your doctor. We strongly recommend you follow his or her advice. Information in this book is general and is offered with no guarantees on the part of the authors or Da Capo Press. The authors and publisher disclaim all liability in connection with the use of this book. The names and identifying details of people associated with events described in this book have been changed. Any similarity to actual persons is coincidental.

Da Capo Press books are available at special discounts for bulk purchases in the U.S. by corporations, institutions, and other organizations. For more information, please contact the Special Markets Department at the Perseus Books Group, 2300 Chestnut Street, Suite 200, Philadelphia, PA, 19103, or call (800) 810-4145, ext. 5000, or e-mail special.markets@perseusbooks.com.

10 9 8 7 6 5 4 3 2 1

# CONTENTS

# INTRODUCTION

## You want to lose weight.

If you're like millions of other people, you've tried and tried. And you've been promised miracles so often you can barely look at the word *diet* anymore without cringing.

You want to look and feel great.

You're tired, you're busy, and you just don't have time to waste. And you certainly don't want to spend hours cooking special foods for yourself on a diet plan. Correct?

You want to be healthy, but not if it takes a huge effort because your energy is already being spent elsewhere.

Well, I don't believe in wasting time—yours or mine. And I don't believe in wasting effort, either. So what I've constructed for you here is a simple plan that is filled with fresh, delicious, whole foods, requires little prep time each day, and will have your body humming with energy before you know it.

*Want to blast off the fat?* Check. You can do that here.

*Want to attain great health?* Check.

*Want to look younger and feel better?* Check and check.

*Want to increase endurance, build lean muscle, and enhance immunity?* Triple check.

And no, I'm not overpromising you a quick fix or selling you a bill of goods. I'll help you prepare the right foods with clean, all natural ingredients, which are packed with many nutrients, plus fat-fighting, immune-boosting abilities. They come straight from plants, trees, and the earth. They are powered by the sun and soil. What's stronger and more powerful than the sun? Our bodies have co-evolved with the plant-life on this planet, and we are designed to eat these foods for maximum benefit. These are the foods our bodies were designed to thrive on day in and day out. These are the foods that blast our energy levels upward and blow away our fat and health issues.

The foods you'll eat on this plan are nature's best fast food. Fast because they require little preparation and no cooking. Just pick them (or pick them up from the shelf of your local farmers' market or super-market), wash them, and they're pretty much ready to go. You'll soon see that the recipes on this plan aren't much more complicated than that.

So how are we going to get from here to there? What will you need to do to send your energy soaring, your health markers positively upward, and your mood, skin, and soon-to-be lean, hot body into the stratosphere?

Over the course of 15 days, we're going to clean out your engine (detoxify) and rebuild your chassis from the inside out (melt off the fat) by filling your tank with special groups of fat-fighting foods that I call Rocket Fuel, so named because they give you a blast of clean energy while they also blast off the pounds.

There are four Rocket Fuel categories, each providing a great weight-loss benefit on its own, but even more powerful when grouped together: probiotics, prebiotics, MCFAs, and thermogenics. You will learn why each is a powerful ally in helping you jettison excess fat and power launching you into the healthiest you possible. Just bring your appetite and your curiosity; I'll supply the rest.

Phase 1, Shake It Up, will detoxify your body and clear out the crud. Even the healthiest of us lives in a fairly toxic environment, and, if you've been eating fake and nutrient-free foods for a long time, you're going to need to clean your engine. Starting clean will give you the best foundation, or launching pad, for achieving maximum weight and fat loss. As this phase's title suggests, shakes and smoothies will be your primary fuel source during these three days. These foods were chosen because of their known detoxification properties and cleansing benefits. And each meal has Rocket Fuels for added boost.

In Phase 2, Melt Down, we'll introduce even more Rocket Fuels but focus in on pro- and prebiotics, as well as MCFAs (a class of fatty acids that are going to be your new BF-FF, best fat-fighting friend). These little food warriors will "eat up" belly fat and other unwanted, unhealthy fat stores.

Phase 3, Blast Off, features meals and recipes designed to contain all four Rocket Fuel groups and to get you to your final goal fast. Every bite benefits you in multiple ways. And your body benefits from the synergistic effects of eating all of the planned meals for this 8-day stretch.

And speaking of eating, my training is as an organic, whole foods chef. Taking nature's gifts and making them into delectable treats is my specialty. And I've done that here in an extensive recipe section. Every meal in the book comes with a super-quick, easy-to-make recipe. (I've even provided options for any of you who want to spend even less time in the kitchen prepping, but we'll talk more about that later.) All recipes have been tested for flavor and effectiveness. Nor will you have to go without dessert on this plan, or feel guilty when you reach for one. All desserts and sweet snacks within the book actually HELP you lose weight and gain health. Fun, huh?

Throughout the book you'll also see little call-out boxes, Power Packed, where I'll highlight one of my personal favorite supercharged foods. Healthy natural multitaskers, these foods will work hard for you. They do the work while you enjoy the benefits.

Once you've finished the 15-day plan, you'll be able to stay in orbit and then later, if you'd like, continue to explore new health realms with my easy tips. Chapter 7, Steady As She Goes, is all about successfully staying on the plan and then later maintaining your weight loss, as well as learning to live your life in a way that keeps you hot, healthy, and energized. Chapter 8, The Next Stage, the final full chapter, is dedicated to helping you take on new challenges and supercharge performance in your now healthier body: you'll learn how to further maximize endurance, build muscle and power, and even increase flexibility.

## SO WHY LISTEN TO ME?

Still need a little convincing? I can understand that. As I said before, you've been promised a lot and have likely received way too little. I've pretty much devoted most of my life to finding ways to eat well—to be healthy and fit, without sacrificing taste. I believe so strongly our health is our most valuable asset, that I've made it my career!

I was raised in the Catskill Mountains of New York, an active child always out in nature. My parents, first generation Koreans, followed and shared with me an extremely healthy diet. They valued gardening and respected the land, and we grew our own organic produce. They also introduced me to juicing and enjoying whole, minimally processed, fresh foods.

With this background, you might think I wouldn't ever have had a weight or health issue. But like so many others, as soon as I was on my own in the first few months of college, I managed to gain about 20 pounds, and my cholesterol skyrocketed to almost 300. This all happened because I was eating processed foods, tons of sugar, deep-fried foods, and loads of white flour, while partying and not exercising like I used to.

When I went home for Thanksgiving that year, my Mom helped snap me back into eating healthy, whole foods that I'd been raised to enjoy. I began to exercise regularly again, and I made my health a priority. And I've done so ever since.

In the early 1990s, I was working and living in the heart of the dot-com boom in San Francisco, and I discovered gourmet raw foods. My first raw dinner fueled my energy, productivity, mental clarity, and gave me laser-like focus. I had a presentation to prepare for the next morning, and I noticed that this dinner had enabled me to stay up all night long, cranking out my multimedia presentation. My focus was so strong; my mind was so clear; and I was hyper-productive. The next morning, my presentation went off without a hitch, and I felt great. Quickly, I realized eating this way also boosted my immune system and kept me from getting sick. Raw food was the perfect tool to help me get through my 100+

hour workweeks. It helped me work faster and more effectively, so I could have time left over for socializing, celebrating, and exercising. I was hooked. What twenty-something wouldn't be?

I began to learn how to prepare raw recipes, and, as I fully embraced a raw food diet, I effortlessly lost an additional 15 pounds in the first month—while stuffing myself at every meal.

I also noticed that allergies I had developed during and after college had all gone away. We had always had dogs when I was a child, but as a young adult, out of the blue, I began getting stuffy, teary-eyed, and I developed itchy hives on my skin whenever I was near an animal. I was so happy that this way of eating eliminated those reactions and I was now no longer allergic to dogs, because I love them so much.

As a competitive child and later varsity athlete (gymnastics, volley-ball, diving, and pentathlon during indoor and outdoor track season) and then as an adult who loved physical exercise (I still think of myself as an athlete, even though I don't compete as much), I'd always been on a quest for fueling my body for optimal peak performance. Now, I was learning how whole, fresh, unprocessed, organic food could fuel the body, mind, and spirit. I carried my own food with me everywhere, and people were intrigued with what I was eating. When they tried it, they liked it. And when I explained the health, mental, physical, and energy benefits, they loved it even more, just like I did. Friends began asking me to bring my dishes to potlucks and parties.

After moving to Los Angeles to consult for a studio designing television and Internet convergence media, my impromptu cooking for these pop-up dinners and events I was hosting and producing as Smart-Monkey Foods® sprouted into a small catering business. It was a way to have delicious, healthy, whole food available to myself and others while I was also working as a Creative Director at the studio. My pop-ups quickly grew to 50 to 100 people every week, and soon, I launched a line of pre-pared packaged foods called SmartMonkey Foods®.

In order to focus on what I loved most, my food business, I decided to relocate to Portland, Oregon, where I helmed workshops, classes, and retreats. I taught raw food prep and nutrition courses and consulted on food fueling for optimal peak performance at Adidas' USA headquarters'

Fitness Center for their athletes and employees, while also providing healthy raw food options at their campus café's and restaurants. I also taught classes at and catered for Whole Foods Markets throughout the Pacific Northwest. I eventually crafted and self-published my *Art of Raw* cookbook, which later grew into *Ani's Raw Food Kitchen*.

Kanga, my Rhodesian Ridgeback, and I found and rescued one another. She weighs about 80 pounds today, but when I adopted her, she was more than 50 pounds underweight, had kennel cough, and was very depressed. Using a raw diet, I healed Kanga back to radiant health over the course of a month or so.

Wanderer and outdoor lover (read: sunshine seeker) that I am, I've since moved back to Los Angeles and written three additional cookbooks: *Ani's Raw Food Desserts*, *Ani's Raw Food Essentials*, and *Ani's Raw Food Asia*. The goal of each of my books is always to inspire readers to include more health-promoting whole foods in their diet, no matter their food preferences.

I want to help people to look and feel their best because from this place, anything is possible!

## WHAT'S IN IT FOR YOU?

I'm on a mission to show everyone how easy, fast, and economical it can be to enjoy delicious, healthy, fresh food and live a healthy lifestyle. It's the biggest and best gift for me when people tell me I've inspired them to change their lives or have even helped save their lives. Following the principles of my past books, many have cleaned up their diets, regained their health, taken control of their lives, and now feel and look great. People have lost significant amounts of weight just by incorporating the recipes from my previous four *uncookbooks* into their daily routine. One person lost 90 pounds in the first year on my raw foods, while many others have told me about healing themselves from illnesses like hypertension, diabetes, and even cancer. I created this detox plan after hearing from so many people who really wanted to try raw foods—for general health, as well as weight loss—but who were intimidated, unsure, or just plain freaked-out by the concept of a raw diet. It's simple; just think of this as a fresh, whole-food diet.

With this plan, people have lost everything from 5 pounds in the first three days to over 80 pounds in a year! And they are keeping it off—with these awesome side effects: radiant skin, more energy and vitality, and increased productivity. Many people have reported that when they continue with the principles of the plan over time, they feel, act, and look younger.

## MODERATION IS KEY—EVEN WHEN GOING RAW

You've probably heard stereotypes about eating raw: it's all raw or nothing and there's no flexibility to it. Well, unlike some others, I don't advocate an all-or-nothing approach. I try to avoid extremes. Health is a lifelong pursuit, and we strive to do better and better each day. I don't want to try being perfect because it's too stressful for me. I don't want you to have that stress, either. Instead, I encourage you to notice how you feel after each adjustment, after each day. This is why I include an interactive, journaling section with each day of the plan, so you can track where you are and how you feel. If you're feeling good, you'll generally keep doing the things that make you feel good. And it works the other way around, too. Feel bad, reach for something that you think is comforting, but ultimately you continue to feel bad.

When you add more fresh, whole foods to your diet, chances are you'll feel lighter, more energetic, stronger, leaner, healthier, and happier. Sometimes, feeling even just a little bit better helps you realize that you weren't feeling so great before. And once you get a taste of how it feels to be strong, vibrant, healthy, and amazing, you will want a bigger bite. Who wouldn't want to feel this great all the time? Then at the next meal or the next day, you strive to do as good or better again, and with each small change, your life and energy blossom. And the move toward optimum health continues. What's not to love?!

So buckle your seat belts and read on because you're in for an enjoyable and healthy ride.

# WHAT TO EXPECT WHEN YOU'RE DETOXING

If you're used to eating a lot of processed foods and heavy meat and dairy dishes, you're going to be amazed at how good you feel when you start eating more whole, fresh veggies and fruits. And . . . you may also initially feel some discomfort. When you start anything new, be it eating, exercise, heck, even a new job, you have to adjust. With adding new foods into your way of eating, your body will need some time to adjust, so you could experience some symptoms of withdrawal. Yes, withdrawal. Processed foods, sugary foods, and the like can be addictive. As new research shows: "Sugary foods and drinks, white bread and other processed carbohydrates that are known to cause abrupt spikes and falls in blood sugar appear to stimulate parts of the brain involved in hunger, craving and reward, the new research shows. The findings, published in The American Journal of Clinical Nutrition, suggest that these so-called high-glycemic foods influence the brain in a way that might drive some people to overeat."

So when you cut these foods out of your diet, what happens? Your body says, "What? Where's the usual stuff?" and as a result, you may feel cruddy at first with the following symptoms:

headache
fatigue
mental fogginess
intense cravings

## Raw Food Feasting vs. Juice Fasting

Raw food is the original, healthy, whole food detox. You can enjoy nutritious and delicious shakes, soups, salads, pastas, burgers, pizzas, and even pies and cakes—seriously—while enjoying the benefits of detoxing. Raw food feasting sounds so much more inviting than starving for days on a juice fast. Green juices are Nature's perfect multivitamin and are great to add into any diet. Yet while we'd never consider only eating multivitamins and foregoing food, people will starve themselves for days on a juice fast. Since we are designed to eat food, juice fasts can create myriad issues. Sure, you might lose a few pounds in water weight, but juice fasts are just another type of crash diet. Your body will go into starvation panic mode and cannibalize its muscle mass, and you can permanently slow down your metabolism.

Of course, no one wants to feel like crap, especially on the quest to get healthy. Like I said earlier, moderation is key. When you're getting ready to start the 15-day plan, you may want to spend a few days or weeks prior reducing your caffeine intake and introducing more veggies into your diet in order to make your transition into the plan as smooth as possible. Here are some ideas:

## BUZZ KILL

The plan allows you to drink all the green tea and water you like; for maximum fat blast, though, you'll need to say no to coffee, alcohol, and sodas (yes, even diet sodas). Green tea has caffeine in it, but if you're used to three triple venti lattes before 8 a.m., you're in for a shock—especially if you go cold turkey. Try to reduce your caffeine intake before the plan; an easy way to do it is to ease into half-decaf drinks and then swap over to green tea. Do you love a dairy bomb in your coffee? Try half soy or almond milk.

## EAT MORE PLANTS

Yep, Michael Pollan said it best: "Eat food. Not too much. Mostly plants." To prep yourself for your blast off, spend the week before incorporating more fruits and veggies into your diet. It can be as simple as swapping out one dairy- or meat-based meal per day. Used to having a hamburger for lunch? Try a veggie burger. Easy changes to your meals include adding fresh fruit to your breakfast or as a snack and adding greens to lunch or dinner (think salad or a handful on your sandwich or as a base for your protein). Raw veggies can be a great snack, too.

## GET YOUR BODY MOVING

This diet is effective without exercise, but we both know that you can't be truly healthy if you sit on your bum all day. All you need is a brisk 20-minute walk daily to get your blood circulating and your heart pumping. Stretching is also beneficial; it will keep healthy oxygen flowing to all the cells in your body to help jettison deeply lodged fat and toxins out of your system.

## REMEMBER WHY YOU'RE DOING THIS

You're reading this book because you want to look and feel better. Investing in your health is one of the best things you can do for yourself (and your friends and family!). So, to put it bluntly: be nice to yourself. Get plenty of rest. Remember that this is a journey.

# PREPARING FOR TAKEOFF

# 1

# THE RAW TRUTH

If you're checking out this plan as a fast way to reboot your system back to a clean, healthy body (just like when you were born) and shed some pounds along the way, you've come to the right place. The foods you'll eat will be fresh, healthy, nutrient-rich, and calorie slim. This means you'll have to eat a lot on this plan. If you're like me, that won't be a chore.

If you want to, you can get started right now on the detox plan. Yes, you can skip this chapter and jump ahead to the diet plan, menus, and recipes. Hey, this is your book, your guide, and it's your choice how you use it. But if you're curious about the philosophy behind the program, and you want to know a little more on why we're both eating this way, then sit down and hang out for a bit and I'll explain. A little later on in the book, if you find you like this natural style of eating, I'll show you how to modify the plan for a healthy, delicious lifestyle all year long.

If you're new to the concept of plant-based, whole, fresh, and uncooked foods, you might think it all seems a little bit "out there," or at least a little unusual. And I bet you think it's really hard to do, too. I can tell you with great certainty, that neither is true, and eating this way is as natural as breathing, once you get the hang of it.

Let's start with the basics: what are raw foods?

## THE GIVEN DEFINITION OF 'RAW'

Raw foods are uncooked, unprocessed, often times organic, and consist of whole foods from nature (not a factory) like fruits, vegetables, nuts, seeds, and sometimes even sprouted grains, dairy, or meat that has not been heated above 118 degrees. Raw foodists don't heat above this temperature because heat is known to lower the nutritional benefits of certain foods while softening plant and other fibers and also releasing water.

## MY DEFINITION OF RAW—
## AND HOW IT WILL BENEFIT YOU

Think of it this way—we have used raw materials, like stones for example, for thousands of years to craft long-lasting buildings (many of which still stand in cities all over the world) and structures (like the Pyramids in Egypt). Sand, thatch, wood, mud, slate, granite, and metals are all still used throughout the world as building materials. I want to help you build something else: a better body and a healthier, more vibrant life.

As I told you in the Introduction, I eat this way—a huge variety of plant foods in their most natural state—so that I can enjoy vibrant health and vitality. There are also some pretty great side effects like gorgeous skin, a lean body, and peak physical and mental performance. If you join me on this journey, your food might not be hot, but you will be! The living foods you'll eat on this plan are replete with vitamins, minerals, and enzymes, vitally important nutrients for optimal health and weight maintenance.

The idea behind eating unprocessed whole fruits, vegetables, nuts, and seeds in their natural and unheated state is that they are packed full of everything a body needs and, because of evolution, easily absorbed by our bodies and familiar to our cells and organs. By avoiding the use of heat, we actually get more bang for our buck (and our utility bills) and more nutrients in every bite. In this book, though, we will use a high-speed blender to "chew" some of our food for us. Why? The blender breaks down food into easily digestible pieces. Drinking many of our meals, especially during Phase 1, means our digestive system doesn't have to work as hard, which, in turn, leaves us with extra energy for detoxing, shedding fat, healing, and fighting illness. This phase alone will go a long way toward helping you reboot and come back to the healthy body you were born with or had just a few short months, or years, ago.

In addition to providing more value from each bite, enjoying whole, clean foods helps us avoid eating dangerous chemicals that are used in manufacturing and processing such as artificial colors, flavors, preservatives, and pesticides (which is why I suggest choosing organic whenever possible). More on fake foods in a minute.

My raw food consists of fruits, vegetables, nuts, and seeds, and I avoid legumes, grains, gluten, and animal products. If heating foods, as in dehydrating, I keep my ingredients below 104 degrees. While some agree on 118 degrees, I choose to heat only to 104 degrees because I believe there's less nutrient loss. (Dehydrating simulates sun drying, and drying food is a good way to extend shelf life, while also creating new textures, like the crunch of a flax cracker.) Raw food is nutritionally dense and naturally detoxifying and cleansing due to its water and fiber content.

Eating and living raw is much more than just a diet. It's a lifestyle that helps us tread lightly on our planet while feeding our body the highest quality fuel available for optimal health and vitality. It's about eating clean and unprocessed foods like our grandparents did, before all the packaged, processed, factory-created junk foods were invented.

Those junk foods, by the way, have been deliberately engineered so that you'll crave more and more of them. How's this for an eye-opener? Michael F. Jacobson of the Center for Science in the Public Interest, wrote a shocking piece for the *Huffington Post* in mid-2011 titled "Coca-Cola's Anniversary: Why I'm Not Celebrating" in which he revealed that we get more calories from soda than food! In his words, "Today, 'liquid candy'— nondiet carbonated soft drinks—is the single largest source of American calories, providing about 7 percent of calories." Nature has no such designs on your pocketbook or on "hooking" you on its product.

I used to be militant about being 100 percent raw. But, in recent years, my experience and path have changed. When it's cold outside, and I'm craving a warm soup, I'll heat up my blended raw soup on the stove in a saucepan, or leave it blending a while to heat it up, or even add hot water to the container when blending. Even though heat damages some nutrients and softens fiber, at least I know that the soup was made with whole, fresh ingredients. My heated raw soup is clean and free of toxic pesticides, preservatives, artificial flavors, and colors. Compared to a can or box of factory-manufactured soup, there's no question what's healthier for me or for you!

The recipes in this book are designed to be enjoyed immediately. They also store and travel well if you're taking them to work or school with you. If it's cold out, and you're craving a hot drink or soup, by all means, heat up your recipe on the stove. To keep it raw, use your finger to test the temperature. As soon as it gets warm to the touch (again that's about 104 degrees), remove your food from the stove and enjoy.

My recipes are vegan, and no matter your food style, it is a good idea to give our bodies a break from certain foods from time to time. If you're an omnivore, I encourage striving to eliminate animal products during this program for optimal results. If you choose to incorporate animal products during the rest of your life, however, I encourage you to seek out healthier options—you'll see suggestions for these later on in the book.

## ☆ POWER PACKED: *Apple Cider Vinegar*

Is cholesterol a problem for you? Are you struggling with insulin control? If either of these is an issue for you, take a peek at the list below. Animal studies have shown that consuming apple cider vinegar can lead to:

- Decreased triglyceride and VLDL (a particularly bad molecule of bad cholesterol) levels in the blood
- Better glucose control in diabetic patients

Among its other benefits, cider vinegar:

- Is a good source of potassium (important for heart function) and calcium (strong bones and weight-control)
- Is fermented, so it contains valuable probiotics. Why should you care? You'll soon learn that probiotics are friendly 'Bots that zip around to eat up our belly fat!

Besides tasting good, apple cider vinegar is commonly used in home remedies:

- As a sunburn cure: mix some in a bath of warm water or soak a washcloth in it and apply locally

- To reduce the symptoms of diarrhea because the pectin in apples is a binder. But don't overdo it: try ½ teaspoon to 1 teaspoon in water to start. (Always consult your doctor before trying this, just in case the problem is more than a case of food disagreeing with you.)

## DON'T GET BOXED IN

One other thing: none of the foods on this plan are pretend-healthy, boxed-up, organic, fake foods. I'm sure almost anyone paying attention to the rising rates of illness and obesity in our culture knows of the massive amount of research pointing to one major culprit: fake, overly processed, nutrient-void, chemical-enriched foods. And sadly, there are many "healthy" versions of this fake food that we are gobbling up. There is no bait and switch with raw.

Raw foods have not been manipulated into unidentifiable forms. They don't have added nutrients. Our bodies know what to do with real foods; as a species, we have eaten them for thousands of years. We know what blueberries are; we recognize cucumbers or pears. But our bodies have a harder time with getting nutrition from things like monosodium glutamate, hydrolyzed proteins, and hydrogenated fats. These foods don't communicate the right messages to our bodies.

What do you want to tell your body? Do you want to send a signal of good health, vibrancy, and well-being? Or would you rather confuse it by putting in all these unnatural, foreign food-like items? The more we manipulate our foods—stripping out nutrients, playing with genetic modification, spraying them with toxins—the more unrecognizable these substances are to our bodies and the sicker we become.

And a word to those of you who still might be saying, "I eat only organic, vegan products. I'm healthy." My response to that is this: what's on your plate? If most of your calories are coming out of a box, you are still eating processed, chemical-laden foods instead of the vegetables and whole foods your body needs and recognizes. What's in the ingredient list for that vegan, organic, nonfood? Pick up your favorite packaged "health" food and read its label. How many ingredients are there? How many of them are unrecognizable as food? How many of them are just plain unrecognizable? Pass the natural sodium phosphate, please. May I have some more monocalcium phosphate and datem? Sorry, but this isn't food. Not real food.

Again, it costs a lot to process, manufacture, market, advertise, and distribute foods. In this equation, not much money is left over for actual "food" ingredients in most processed foods. There's room for fillers, preservatives, chemicals, and lots of wheat and corn byproducts, but there's not much left for the actual whole food.

I can tell you that even manufacturers with the best of intentions aren't going to give you in a box something that nature can: a diet that is full, replete, and rich with flavor and nutrients, as well as immune-boosting and anti-aging power. And those with the worst intentions (read David Kessler's, *The End of Overeating* to find out how food companies prey on our addictions to sugar, salt, and fat in creating the foods they do) will sink your health in a minute in pursuit of profit.

## EVEN MORE RAW TRUTHS

There are many myths surrounding eating a living, whole foods diet, especially about meals that aren't processed with heat (cooked). But what's so strange about not cooking, really? And for those of you who hate to cook, why wouldn't you fully embrace this way of eating?

If you think about it for more than a microsecond, you'll discover that you already enjoy raw foods and probably more than just a few foods in this state. How would you answer any of these questions? Grabbed an apple, orange, or a pear to snack on? Eaten salsa and guacamole? Snacked on sashimi or a salad? Is a carrot, apple, or salad weird or strange? (It may be that you haven't enjoyed salads yet, but I bet you'll change your mind once you've tried some of my salad recipes.)

If you're still feeling a little doubtful or think this is wacky, boring, or too hard, let me share some more truths.

## RAW TRUTH #1: THE FOOD TASTES DELICIOUS

I can prove my point pretty quickly on this one. Ever sit outside on a sunny day and eat a ripe peach or a slice of watermelon? Does anything taste better? (And don't say chocolate cake, unless you're talking about my Chocolate Raspberry Ganache, which my editor—an avowed cake-a-holic but lazy baker—says is awesome. Her kids like it, too. Their new favorite is my chocolate lava cakes. You can find the recipe for both in *Ani's Raw Food Desserts*.)

Real food tastes really good. It's that simple.

If you're used to eating foods from a package, you'll be both surprised and delighted by the variety of tastes available in this diet and lifestyle. Yummy and mouth-watering fruit smoothies, delicious soups and salads, great wraps, rolls, noodles, meals—and even desserts and sweet snacks! Once you've taken a break from overly processed, packaged foods, you'll discover that your taste buds won't like them so much. You'll actually taste the chemicals and fakeness when you try them again. They won't taste nearly as good to you because you'll have trained your body to want the real stuff, and you'll taste the delicious difference.

After you've completed the plan, I challenge you to try your favorite junk food side-by-side with one of the amazing desserts offered here. Let me know who wins. I already know the answer, and so do you!

## RAW TRUTH #2: YOU EAT A TRUCKLOAD OF FOOD

Okay, it may not be humanly possible, or even desirable, to eat quite this much. The point I'm truly making here is that this plan is designed to have you eating whenever you're hungry and as much of the foods on the plan as you'd like.

You don't have to starve yourself thin. You don't have to deprive yourself thin. You don't have to count calories. You don't have to worry about any of this. You don't have to do anything other than to eat what nature intended for you: delicious, fresh, clean, health-promoting food!

Let's talk about portions for a moment. I don't believe in portion control. Humans love to eat. It's built into our DNA. Many diet plans forget this basic concept and are so restrictive that followers are almost set up to fail before they begin. If you're eating a high volume of the right foods, the Rocket Fuels, you can't go wrong. Eat a ton of the processed, nutrient-devoid foods I talked about earlier and your health goes south, your fat stores grow, and not much of anything good can come of it.

## RAW TRUTH #3: FOOD IS ACTUALLY *EASIER* TO MAKE

Busy? Tired? Stressed? Join the club; we've got millions of members. Many of us are eternally running to keep up with the daily demands of our lives. Preparing meals seems like just one more thing on your I-don't-want-to-do list on busy days and on most diet plans.

Maybe you are one of those people who just doesn't like to cook at all, or maybe you're someone who doesn't mind doing it, but you feel unskilled or just not good at it. Well, wherever you sit, I've got good news: you don't have to cook at all! Plus, you can learn how to mix, blend, and match foods so they taste amazing and deliver the most health punch. How's that for a good benefit package? And you get a daily bonus, too, in that the clean-up is a snap because nothing is baked, cooked, or dried on. Nothing has to be scraped, scoured, or worked over to use again. Just rinse your utensils and equipment and voila! Clean, clean, clean.

Tired of slaving over a stove at the end of a long day trying to follow the latest new diet? Well, now you don't have to because you'll use a blender or food processor for most meals. Often all you have to do is dump some great foods into a pitcher or bowl, press a button, and you're done. Most preparation you'll have to do on any given day won't add up to more than rinsing off and cutting up some produce. Nature has already supplied the best fast foods there are, with no drive-thru needed.

I'll get you started with shopping lists—so a trip to the super-market or farmers' market will be fast and painless—as well as provide you with a short list of basic tools and pantry items to keep on hand over the next weeks. Don't worry; we won't break the bank buying lots of equipment and items you'll never use again. You won't need anything fancier than a blender.

I don't want to make losing weight and getting healthy difficult. We want it to be simple, satisfying, and delicious. I'll give you all the tools you need; it's up to you what you do with them. If you want to see the maximum benefits, I urge you to try the full 15-day plan. I designed it to blast off the pounds fast and improve your health. But if you want to just try it for a day? Go ahead. Want to skip around? Do so. But do try the plan and this way of eating. I promise you'll be happy with how it makes you feel and look.

## RAW TRUTH #4: FOOD IS FASTER TO PREPARE

I've a pretty simple question for you that may help you decide if this plan is for you. What would you prefer to do? Would you rather spend hours or minutes in the kitchen? If you answered hours, then you are likely a serious foodie who loves to prep, cook, and spend any free time you have in the kitchen. I get that. It's my favorite place to be, too. I'm a chef after all! But if you're like so many time-strapped, overworked people, you want to be in and out of there as fast as possible. And this book gives you that option.

I've constructed each recipe to be super simple, very fast (minutes, not hours, in the kitchen), and with easy cleanup. I don't believe you should feel like you're wasting time in your life or in your kitchen; there's too much else to do, enjoy, and explore.

Many cookbooks promise 30-minute meals. Even though I think that's a relatively short time to spend in the kitchen (I love to play with my food all day long!), none of your meals in this plan will take nearly that long. Sometimes you can whip together these dishes in seconds, and often in a mere handful of minutes.

Many people ask me if you can go gourmet and still eat raw. Absolutely. All the recipes provided here are delectable and creatively spiced. But going gourmet isn't really what this plan is all about. I want you sleek, healthy, beautiful, and energized—without spending all your free hours in the kitchen.

## RAW TRUTH #5:
## REAL FOOD IS CHEAPER, MORE ECO-NOMICAL™

One of the first questions I often hear about eating real, whole foods is this: isn't it expensive? Even though they may cost more than a dollar-meal at a local fast food eatery or some pre-packaged "death" foods, I believe that these foods are highly eco-nomical™. What do I mean by that?

Well, if your goal is to look great, let's do the math. Instead of spending hundreds of dollars on dermatologic procedures, antiwrinkle regimens, and expensive skincare products that contain limited amounts of the nutrients (like vitamin C) and antioxidants known to help skin, why not build better skin to begin with by "applying" these substances to your insides? Eat the foods that create clean, clear, radiant skin; internally treat and nourish your cells, not topically, and your skin will thank you for it. Your skin is your largest organ, and feeding it right just makes good sense and is more effective—and more cost-effective— than multiple trips each year to the dermatologist for injections and procedures.

You have to eat, right? So why not spend your money on great health-boosting food, instead of trips to the doctor, aesthetician, or drugstore? Would you rather apply some chemicals that have been sitting on a shelf for over a year or feed your skin straight from nature? How enjoyable can surgery, supplements, and injections be? Not!

I won't say that whole foods are inexpensive; sadly, that's not the case. But organic, local, or regional produce is becoming more widely available, and as more people switch to eating this way, the costs will go down. And while you may have to spend more out of pocket initially, the costs are so much less than continuing down your current path. The benefits to your health, vitality, and longevity far outweigh the added expense.

It's not just good for you, though. Eating this way is ecologically economical (why I say eco-nomical™ above). It's better for the planet in both the long and short terms. Food doesn't have to travel thousands of miles, so fuel costs and emissions are reduced. Because these foods are grown locally and organically, they aren't sprayed with chemicals to make them look good, as well as toxins and pesticides. You ingest fewer of these unnatural and often poisonous substances, and the Earth doesn't have to swallow them either.

## RAW TRUTH #6: YOU WILL BE BLOAT-FREE

This one ruffles my feathers because people think eating fresh, whole foods leaves you gassy, bloated, and uncomfortable. Not true. Common food allergens include dairy, wheat, gluten, refined sugar, and animal products. That means eating them will cause an immune response and inflammation, or swelling. So when we decrease or eliminate foods that make us bloat up, we shrink down and lean out. I also avoid legumes (never eat raw legumes because they are toxic; eat only cooked legumes), which are hard to digest and are known to cause gas and bloating. By eating my Rocket Fuels, the fat-fighting, multitasking health warriors you'll read more about soon, you'll be automatically decreasing this unwanted side effect.

Combine too little fiber and too little activity, and guess what you get? Constipated and bloated. And guess how you'll look? Not so hot. Eat too fast, and you'll also add to the bloat because you're not chewing your foods enough to aid your digestive system (more on that in a minute). Instead, you are stressing it. Artificial sweeteners and sodium are also culprits in bloating. Guess what you avoid with raw foods? Yep, those nasty foods that need to be loaded with both in order to taste good. Our food tastes good naturally.

We don't just actively avoid foods that will bloat us. We embrace foods that are bloat-fighters in this plan: probiotics, fermented foods, ginger, and pineapple, to name just a few.

As I first shared in my book, *Ani's Raw Food Kitchen*, I lost 15 pounds during my first month of eating only fresh whole organic foods every day. And I was stuffing myself! But the water and fiber I was filling up on were sweeping all my cells clean; I let go of stored toxins and fat, and my fat cells shrank. You can experience this, too. You'll see the results very quickly, which is a great motivator to keep you trekking on down this new path a little longer.

And there's another bonus: the desserts I've created on this diet will not hurt you (health-wise or fat-wise); they'll actually HELP you lose more weight. So forget this common misconception. You'll be a lean, green-eating, gorgeous, and happy machine—tanked up, not swelled up, with all the good stuff you'll eat.

## RAW TRUTH #7: FOOD IS EASIER TO DIGEST

One of the key reasons that food on this plan is easier to digest is because of simple ingredients and simple foods. You'll eliminate many of the common allergens—like wheat, soy, dairy—which tax the digestive system. You will have better digestion, better assimilation, and better elimination, too.

I ask you to refrain from eating all animal proteins—meats, eggs, milk, fish—for the duration of the plan. I'm also going to ask that you stay away from wheat products. Most of us rely too heavily on wheat in our daily diets. This over-reliance pushes out other nutrient-rich foods from the diet. Even those who don't have Celiac sprue can still experience irritation and inflammation if they are sensitive to wheat. I want you to eat the cleanest food possible for the next 15 days. Not only to clean out your engines, but also to rebuild your insides from a cellular level. And as I'm sure you suspect from the heading of this section, one of the most important systems we'll tune up is your gut.

I mentioned that this plan will focus on foods that help with bloating, but the plan goes a little further than that. I want to help you create the best and most smoothly running intestinal tract you can have. The healthier it is, the healthier you are. The foods you'll eat here increase healthy flora and beneficial bacteria. With the right balance in your intestines, you'll have a few trillion more friends on your side in your weight-loss battle.

### ✿ A Cure for IBS?

Penni Shelton, a lifelong IBS (irritable bowel syndrome) sufferer, is the force behind www.RawFoodRehab.ning.com. If you're suffering from IBS, it might be well worth reading what she has to say.

"Within one week of switching to a diet of raw and living foods, ALL of my symptoms of IBS were gone! As you might imagine, I was in shock, amazed, and totally sold on this unbelievably simple new way of eating. Besides the intestinal relief, I lost 15 pounds in the first month, and over the past five years, my overall health and well-being has continued to improve.

"I've found that foods in their natural state are much easier for my body to process and eliminate, which I believe is the key to why eating this way has had such a dramatic healing effect on treating my IBS. I know I'm not alone as I have seen these same kinds of experiences in thousands of people worldwide."

Also, you'll be eating what Nature intended for you to eat: foods that humans have evolved with, so our bodies recognize them and know what to do with them. There is no guess work for it to puzzle through, like when identifying fake fats and odd byproducts. These are foods we were designed to eat.

I mentioned Rocket Fuel a few pages ago, and if you've followed me in other books, you've heard me say this before. Most of what we eat is anything but! What's amazing is that the human body is able to run on the lowest grade fuel. Imagine how much that takes away from the overall quality of life and health of the vehicle. But cleaner, purer fuels burn better; put these in your engine and everything runs more smoothly. Which would you rather put in your tank?

## RAW TRUTH #8: CALORIES *DON'T* EQUAL ENERGY

If you are used to feeling sluggish and exhausted, you're not alone. And yes, if you've been reading this chapter closely you know what I'm about to say. It's the food you're eating! You think you need foods that are *calorie*-dense, so you can take on the world and be raring to go. But nope, that's just not true. You need foods that are *nutrient*-dense, and you'll get more than your fair share of those on this plan. What do I mean by nutrient-dense? Simply that a food is rich in nutrients while not packed with calories (because there are no empty calories or fillers); it's the ratio of "goodies" inside a food to the number of calories it contains. These foods are slim on calories and heavy with nutrition.

So many people suffer under a misconception that is hurting their health and their energy levels: calories consumed equals energy felt. I'll prove that equation wrong pretty simply right now. Ever been hit by that afternoon energy dip that knocks you down around 3 pm? And what did you do? Did you grab some chips, a soda, some candy? How did you feel afterward? I'll bet it went something like this: you ate it and felt good for about 20 minutes, but then you felt hungrier and more tired than ever. Yes?

Reaching for that snack or treat that is loaded with salt, sugar, fat, and lots of calories will not do more than give you a momentary boost. Why? Most of those foods have been stripped of actual nutrients or never had them to begin with. They weren't designed to meet your nutritional needs, just to fire up your tastebuds. They have good mouth feel, and you'll want to eat more of them.

We are more than the sum of the calories we consume each day. You've heard it before, but the quality of those calories really counts. Grab sugary, salty crap food and you'll feel a little rush, sure, but then you'll drop like a stone, both in energy and mood, because these foods are devoid of the nutrition—vitamins, enzymes, nutrients—that really lift you up. Eat this way regularly and you'll likely be hungry all the time (wanting more to eat, with every bite, rather than feeling sated) and be getting fatter and unhappier with each added pound. Not to mention that these foods are addictive (really), so you'll just want to keep eating them. "You can't eat just one" is actually a scary truth—one that diminishes your health and increases your waistline.

You'll have tons of energy with raw foods because your body will be getting a truckload's worth of nutrients, rather than a thimbleful. Yes, you may end up eating fewer calories on this plan, but you will be eating more food and all of it will count.

Fewer calories + richer, nutrient-filled foods = a highly energized, super-hot you.

## RAW TRUTH #9: REAL FOOD IS FRIENDLIER AND HEALTHIER—ESPECIALLY FOR FOOD SENSITIVES

I briefly mentioned earlier that this way of eating avoids some of the most common food allergens: wheat, dairy, gluten, and soy. But it's also animal-friendly and cruelty-free. You won't have to search for cage-free, pasture-fed, or any other of the terms meant to ease your mind or conscience when eating animal proteins. If you're not interested in going full-on vegetarian or vegan, that's your choice to make. Again, this is your life, your diet, and only you can decide what feels best for you. On the other hand, choosing to decrease or eliminate animal products means animals are not harmed, which is extra karma bonus points. So why not try a completely different way of eating for these two weeks plus? It's good for the planet; it's good for you; and our little animal friends will appreciate it, too.

If you decide afterward that you can't live without animal proteins, I recommend choosing those that come straight from Mother Earth, like organic grass-fed beef or bison (for lower saturated fat and higher protein content). Avoid mass factory-farmed meats that are full of poisonous antibiotics and other dangerous chemicals and raised and processed in scary ways. A recent study of grocery store shelves found that over 50 percent of the meats tested had staph bacteria in them. Yuck!

## RAW TRUTH #10:
## IT'S YOUR DIET, AND YOU ARE IN CONTROL

I can't state strongly enough how much I'd like for you to at least try to follow the 15-day plan exactly as I've written it. I feel this so strongly because I know just what a world of good it will do for you. I've been living, thriving, on this way of eating for years.

You'll see that in Chapter 7, Steady As She Goes, I mention animal proteins and nonraw items in some of the lists provided. Please note, these are NOT part of the basic plan; you won't see them in any of the recipes I provide to guide you through the next couple of weeks. But if eating these foods is something you feel you need to do, or something you just choose to do, I've provided the best choices from what's available in the scientific literature for your long-term success.

It's your diet. Your life. Your plan. How you live it is up to you. So many people get derailed when they can't stick to the letter of a diet or lifestyle that they just give up and throw in the towel. They go back to the same bad patterns that led them to needing to shed extra pounds. Instead of being realistic with themselves about what their own unique tastes and needs are, they blame themselves or the diet. As a result, they'll try a new plan and another new plan and experience the same troubled waters each time. And so the ripple of ill health continues unstopped.

I know this way of eating is what's best for our bodies. You need to know it, feel it, and believe it for yourself. Take ownership of it and make it your own. If that means your lifestyle differs slightly from mine, that's okay. If you're making an effort to eat more whole, live, plant-based foods, you'll be doing your body a world of good in the long run.

## DRAGGING OR PURRING? IT'S YOUR CHOICE

We have gotten so far away from the experience of whole, nourishing foods, that we don't even know how best to eat them. We buy the most popular brand or the one we think sounds or looks the healthiest. But if you do just one thing differently in your day, do this: Avoid brandname foods because they often won't have much food in them, or very little that a body needs to function well. That's because the makers of branded foods spend most of their money on marketing to ensure that you'll recognize their brand across regions, nations, and the entire world. The name of a branded food remains the same even when language changes.

What you'll eat on this plan, even just by trying 15 days of this diet, will give you the needed rocket fuel to blast through even the most difficult of days.

Do you want to be a hot, well-oiled machine? Energy on high, purring and moving sleekly through your life? Or are you content to drag along, sputtering and puttering through each day? I don't think any of us would deliberately choose sputtering and puttering, but so often that's what we do because of the foods we ingest.

If you really think about what you're putting into your body—not for guilt, not for stress—because you want to take good care of yourself, then it truly is simple. The Raw Food Detox will reintroduce you to flavor-rich, nutrient powerhouses: real food! Say goodbye to tasteless junk that has no benefit, and revel in how good you feel and look. Try it on for size. What do you have to lose (except unwanted excess pounds)? You'll gain so much, including spending less time worrying about what you're not doing right and how you're not caring for yourself and more time in your life doing the fun things you want to do.

If you want to dig deeper into the other health benefits of this diet and lifestyle, then get ready. That's what's coming up next.

# 2

# READY . . .
# WHAT'S IN IT FOR YOU?

You've picked up this book, which tells me you're entertaining the idea of committing to this program for the next 15 days. You might be secretly thinking, why should I change what I do? It's too much effort to try yet another diet that won't work, or work for long. Well, after almost two decades of eating this way and having people constantly asking me how to eat healthier, I wanted to develop a program that would make learning how to eat more whole, unprocessed, fresh foods very simple. My passion is helping people look and feel their best.

In the last chapter, I told you the truth about this style of eating, certainly. But what if you think you'll need more motivation than that to stick with it? That's the aim of this chapter: sharing the wealth of health goodies that come along with following the Raw Food Detox so that you'll be able to refer back here whenever you need a reminder to stick with the journey.

When you eat the foods I'll "prescribe" for you, you'll immediately see and feel the difference. Nutrient-rich foods instantly give your body a boost, like giving a car a jumpstart, which will help you get the most out of each day. And with our busy lives, who doesn't want (or need) to do that? Long term, though, you'll gain stamina, endurance, mental clarity, focus, productivity—all things I have in abundance since I began eating this way. My friends call me the Energizer Bunny because I'm so active and productive, always hopping from new project to new project, while also playing hard. If you want this type of enthusiasm and energy, keep reading. These are great bonuses, and you won't have to rely on your boss to give them to you! I've made it easy for you. Promise.

## BONUS #1: LOSE WEIGHT

Okay, this is a little bit of a cheat, as most of you are coming to the plan just for this purpose. But you can and will lose weight following this plan. There is a huge body of research supporting the many health benefits of a plant-based diet, and one of those well-known benefits is weight control.

Many people have successfully lost weight on other raw diets, yet I've had terrific success with those who specifically followed the Raw Food Detox plan. One early adopter was delighted to find that he'd lost four pounds in just the first three days. But he's not alone. So many now know that this fast, nutritious way of eating is one of the simplest methods to use to watch the pounds evaporate.

Angela Stokes is a great example. This author of *Raw Emotions* and the website www.RawReform.com was morbidly obese at almost 300 pounds. She lost over 160 pounds and made this style of eating her life's passion; now she lectures, consults, blogs, and inspires others to make other transformations in their lives.

One of my favorite stories of extreme weight loss on a natural foods diet comes from Philip McCluskey, www.philipmccluskey.com. Let his words inspire you.

> I stepped on the scale one day and realized that I weighed 400 lbs, and something needed to be done quickly if I was going to live much longer. I was reading a book about fasting and saw the words *raw food* and just felt like it was calling to me. I ordered a bunch of books and dove right in, changing my life overnight. Switching to a raw food lifestyle has changed every area of my life. Not only have I lost over 215 lbs— and kept it off for over three years—I also noticed increased confidence, spirituality, and a general overall improvement of the joy and happiness in my life.

A basic, raw diet is one of the most effective tools there is for shedding weight and improving health. And plant-based diets in general are the healthiest ones around. There's plenty of evidence out there to support this statement. I could write a whole book on it, even. But because terrific sources already exist, and I don't want to write a whole book on the subject, I'll point you to two of the best experts around: Dr. Caldwell Esselstyn and John Robbins. Dr. Esselstyn, a noted heart surgeon on a mission to reverse heart disease, has written of the numerous beneficial effects of eating a vegan diet. He advocates for this way of eating based on the results of a 20-year nutritional study he conducted. If you want to know more, read his book, *Prevent and Reverse Heart Disease*, or go to his website, www.heartattackproof.com. Or you can review *The Food Revolution: How Your Diet Can Help Save Your Life and Our World* by John Robbins (of Baskin Robbins fame: the ice cream empire's heir who turned vegan). If a whole book's not for you, visit his blog www.johnrobbins.info.

The longest-lived people on earth eat simply and live simply. Their diets are chock full of real, unprocessed foods and plenty of plants in their natural states. They are not ingesting chemicals, pesticides, antibiotics, or growth hormones—clean, real food. There's nothing cleaner than food in its rawest state (after washing off the dirt, that is) and nothing better for trimming your waistline.

But this plan steps beyond a basic raw diet like the one Angela and Philip followed, already effective for weight loss, by supercharging it with some additional fat-fighting weapons that you'll read about in the next chapter. You'll also learn about three short phases that will quickly blast away the pounds, toxins, and excess fat.

Check out Philip's five favorite tips for weight loss. They'll help you experience continued success along your journey.

## Philip McCluskey's
## Top Five Weight-Loss Tips

**WATER.** Drink water daily, and eat lots of high-water-content foods like cucumbers, celery, and leafy greens. (Among its other benefits, water fills you up. It's better to reach for these when you're hungry because often we confuse hunger for thirst.)

**GREENS.** Be sure to include a green juice or a smoothie at least once a day. It's a great meal replacement and will help you take in massive amounts of greens. (This doesn't mean a sugar-filled, junk-laden jumbo drink, but rather real greens and lean proteins blended from whole foods into a healthy drink.)

**EXERCISE.** Move your body daily, even if it's a simple walk around the neighborhood. Don't be afraid to get your sweat on.

**ATTITUDE.** Be positive; laugh a lot; watch funny movies; say positive affirmations; rediscover your childlike innocence. Life is supposed to be fun!

**BREATHING.** Breathe; stay present and in the moment; let go of all worry and fear. Breathe into your power and know that you are unstoppable.

## BONUS #2: BUILD MUSCLE MASS

The Raw Food Detox diet does not require exercise to work. This isn't to say that I advocate a sedentary life. Rather, I wanted to tackle in this particular section a huge myth about building muscle while eating raw or vegan. It's clear that the more muscle we have, the better our metabolism runs, and the more calories we burn. But if you thought you needed to follow a meat-based diet to build muscle, think again. That's just not true. I'll prove it.

What's the largest, strongest animal you can think of? Don't say your boyfriend or husband. Let's instead take a look at a close relative: the gorilla. What does he or she eat? Vegetation and lots of it. Same for monkeys and rhinos and many other noticeably strong mammals.

All plants contain protein, and eating a wide variety of them will provide your body with what it needs to maintain optimal health. We'll be adding some of the richest sources of these proteins to your plate in the form of sea vegetables, dark green leafies, and spirulina. Buckwheat, nuts, and seeds are other great sources we'll chomp on, as well as hemp (which is a good source of both protein and brain-sharpening, immune-boosting Omega 3s). And while these foods may be completely new to you (I can hear you: spiru-what? buckwhat?), the fact is this is the sort of food we are meant to eat to be lean and strong. I even enjoy brown rice protein powder that is minimally processed and loaded with protein (17 to 23 grams, depending on the brand). It's also light on fat and carbs (only 1 gram of fat and 3 grams of carbs) per 2-tablespoon serving.

You can build muscle on a raw or vegan diet. But muscle doesn't grow itself; you do have to move a bit to help out! If you're not already active, adding some light strength training or calisthenics to your routine is acceptable and a great place to start growing some. Do push-ups and sit-ups, lift weights or use resistance bands, or simply contract your muscles in a focused manner to activate them, hold for a few seconds, then release, and repeat. I like squat thrusts, leap frogs, and lunges that work my thighs and glutes—the largest muscles in the body.

Sweat a little. Cardio won't build huge muscle mass, per se, but it will feel good and get rid of the toxins, help your circulation, infuse oxygen, and burn more calories.

If you don't want to exercise, I'm not going to tell you that you have to do it to lose weight on this plan. The diet doesn't rely on it, as I stated above. You already know you need to move every day. How you do that, again, is up to you and what your lifestyle demands and needs. One more note: on this plan, you won't want to go hard at the gym unless your body is already adjusted to doing it, or if quick weight loss isn't your goal. An increased appetite often comes with beginning hard-core exercise, which can make it a bit more difficult to stick with any diet plan effectively.

Staying on track and staying motivated can be challenging for anyone, at any time, though. We can be our own worst enemies, sometimes, can't we? Robert Cheeke, a prominent vegan bodybuilder and host of www.VeganBodyBuilding.com, gave me some great motivational tips—check out the sidebar below.

## Robert Cheeke's Top Five Muscle-Building Tips

**EAT UP.** Consume more calories than you are expending if you plan to build muscle.

**BE DENSE.** Eat the most nutrient-dense foods and keep whole foods as the foundation of your nutrition program: namely fruits, vegetables, nuts, and seeds.

**FIND YOUR PURPOSE.** Have a meaningful purpose behind your vision to build muscle mass. Why does it matter to you in the first place? Answer that question honestly; acknowledge what it really means to you; and embrace a fitness program with enthusiasm.

**KEEP IT CONSISTENT.** Be consistent with your training and nutrition programs. Nothing leads to failure more than a break in consistency, and nothing leads to greater improvement and success than consistency and true accountability.

**PRACTICE COMPOUND MOVES.** Focus on weight training and performing compound (multijoint) free-weight exercises such as squats, deadlifts, presses, and pulling exercises. Those stimulate the most muscle growth.

For the next two weeks, stick to the strength training and light exercise mentioned above, if you want to get exercise in at all. Once you've blasted off the fat and pounds, check out The Next Stage, a chapter I've crafted for pushing performance to the next level. In the Building Muscle section you'll see tips, information, and recipes for adding muscle and increasing power.

# BONUS #3: INCREASE ENERGY AND ENDURANCE

You already know that the type of fuel you put in your motor affects how well your car drives. It's the same with your health. Are you going for high-octane or leaden, weighted-down fuel? Eating whole, natural foods won't leave you dragging your caboose around, but instead it will fill you with strength and overall vitality.

You'll combine foods in special ways, as well as learn how to hydrate properly, so as to boost your overall endurance. You'll mix protein, fats, sugars, and fiber to ensure you receive the longest burning fuel, so you don't crash at any point in the day. And the foods you'll use are rich with energy-boosting nutrients like B vitamins.

Eating nature's original fast foods will reduce stress on the body, overall because they are filled with stress-fighting antioxidants, vitamins, minerals, and enzymes. Less stress = more energy.

This plan ensures that your body works less hard at digestion. Did you know digestion takes up A LOT of energy and time? It takes on average between 75 to 80 hours to thoroughly digest a food. But if we chew it for you by mixing/blending, you'll be able to absorb the nutrients faster, use less energy in the digestion process, and have more time for the things you want to do in your life.

Less work + more nutrients = more energy.

Let's peek at just one of the many Rocket Fuels in the plan, green tea (we'll look at this and others more closely in the next chapter, but I love this one so much you'll see I've made it a Power Packed selection, too). Green tea has been extensively researched for its many, many health benefits (including its ability to promote fat loss). But did you know it also increases endurance? A 10-week animal study in which green tea extract was administered showed that mice could swim up to 24 percent longer. (To work as an endurance enhancer, though, you have to drink it daily. You won't get these benefits by drinking just a single cup.)

## BONUS #4:
## DEVELOP HEALTHY, RADIANT, GLOWING SKIN

So we've established that you'll lose weight, be stronger, have more energy and endurance. In short, you'll feel great. Guess what else happens? You'll also look amazing.

I cannot tell you how many people comment on my complexion and ask, "What do you do for your skin?" When I tell people my age, they are often surprised. My secret is found in the book in your hands and the information it provides about eating and living. But don't just take my word for it. Read what Tonya Zavasta, author of *Beautiful on Raw*, www.beautifulonraw.com, has to say about transforming your looks through the foods you choose.

> Your skin becomes hydrated and dewy; your eyes shine with a healthy glow; your weight normalizes, stabilizes. When your body becomes cleansed and healthy, you'll have all the energy and enthusiasm you could ever want. And this in itself is an integral part of beauty. For those of us forty and over, beauty really is health. When people can see your health by looking at your clear eyes, flawless complexion, and full, healthy hair, they'll see you as beautiful, and they'll tell you so.

I couldn't have said it better myself.

### Tonya Zavasta's
### Top Beautifying Foods

**LEAFY GREENS.** Kale, romaine, and seaweeds, specifically nori.

**VEGETABLE JUICES.** My favorites are beet root, bok choy, cucumber, zucchini, and apple.

**GREEN SMOOTHIES.** Specifically, those including mango and Swiss chard.

**SOAKED RAW NUTS.** Have a handful of nuts each day. I'm fond of pistachios and walnuts. To soak nuts, submerge them in filtered water for about eight hours then rinse them thoroughly before eating. (We soak them to remove harmful tannic acid and enzyme inhibitors so the nuts become easy to digest while releasing their full nutritional value. Soaking also makes the nut softer and easier to chew, while increasing protein content.)

**LOW-SUGAR FRUITS.** I love green apples, avocado, and blueberries.

You'll get to sample for yourself more of Tonya's fabulous foods later in the book.

## BONUS #5: ENHANCE MENTAL PERFORMANCE

You may not be aware of it, but the average American is at risk for being iodine-deficient. Iodine is a trace mineral that is very important to maintaining healthy thyroid function (important for weight management) and strong mental function, as well. According to the website, www.WorldsHealthiestFoods.com, a terrifically informative source of information on whole foods, "Even a mild iodine deficit in pregnant women, infants, and children can lower intelligence by 10 to 15 IQ points, lessening an individual's mental abilities throughout life."

The good news is this plan contains excellent sources of iodine in the form of vegetables that grow in the ocean like kelp, dulse, hijiki, and nori—great gifts from the sea. If you want to be sure you get enough iodine in your diet, make sea vegetables such as these a staple.

☆ **POWER PACKED:** *Nori*

Sea vegetables like nori (as well as kelp, hijiki, wakame, kombu, and dulse) are some of the top sources of dietary iodine and are staples in my kitchen. Nori has been used for centuries as a weight-loss aid. They are a good source of health-promoting vitamin K and folate, too.

Did you also know that they are an excellent source of most any mineral found in the ocean? Researchers are just beginning to understand the enormous wealth of nutrients and health benefits available from consuming these regularly. What's known now? Nori and other sea vegetables:

- Decrease inflammation in the body and provide benefit to osteoarthritis sufferers
- Act as natural anti-coagulants in the blood, improve total cholesterol levels, and decrease bad (LDL) cholesterol
- May lower the risk of developing colon and breast cancers
- Work with our thyroid to balance the body's hormonal system
- The iodine in sea vegetables is also believed to help fight radiation sickness and heavy metal poisoning.

Nice, huh?

One thing to be aware of, though, is to buy certified organic. These foods, if grown in polluted waters, can become contaminated with heavy metals (such as lead, mercury, and arsenic), elements you don't want to be ingesting if your desire is optimal health.

You'll also find foods that are rich in B vitamins, which may help to fight depression. We'll load your plate with Omega 3s, which help improve brain function (and you'll read in the next chapter why they're also a great weight-loss aid). And we'll pile on folate-rich foods—parsley, broccoli, collards and other greens, cauliflower, spinach, and asparagus—shown to help fight dementia, as well as insomnia and irritability.

## BONUS #6: IMPROVE OVERALL HEALTH

There is a huge amount of research documenting the many benefits of eating a plant-based diet. And even though less scientific review has been done to date on eating raw, because this way of living relies on plants as its biggest source of nutrition, the same benefits do apply.

They include:

- A reduction of risk for many chronic diseases, and, as a result,
- Increased overall longevity
- Lower overall rates of cancer
- Lower risk of dying from heart disease
- Lower incidence of type-2 diabetes
- Lower blood pressure levels
- Lower levels of bad and total cholesterol
- Less body mass (folks get and stay skinnier)

## BONUS #7:
## SLOW AGING AND EXTEND LONGEVITY

Let's go back to the analogy I used earlier about what type of fuel you want to put in your tank. Do you want to eat in a way that rusts the pipes of your engine, clogging up the works and making all your body systems work harder and less efficiently? Or do you want a clean, well-oiled machine? A rusted engine breaks down sooner. A well-cared for vehicle purrs along for a good long time. I've asked it before, but what's your choice going to be?

You've probably heard a lot over the years about antioxidants and how they're important to your health. We know that fruits and veggies are the best sources of these substances. But do you know why scientists say they're good for you? It's because these substances fight the "rusting" inside your arteries and keep them free and clear. Your veins and arteries are your body's interior highways. Do you want them jammed up with traffic or freely moving and doing their job of transporting what's important? Less "traffic" (the oxidants responsible for the rusting) means less wear and tear on your engines and a longer-lived vehicle—one that can take you where you want to go without breaking down!

## BONUS #8: PURGE TOXINS

The liver is the organ in our body that detoxifies us of chemicals. And in our rather toxic world, it is getting worked overtime. If your body doesn't have to fight this environmental onslaught so much, it can have more room to heal, and your immune system becomes stronger. Foods that support the liver's function are key to helping us shed these toxins, as well as our extra pounds.

On this plan we ramp up the foods that can help this important organ perform at its best. They include:

- High fiber, organic fruits and vegetables (avocado, apples, berries, broccoli)
- Sulfur-rich foods (onions and garlic)
- Cruciferous veggies (brussels sprouts, kale, cabbage, collards)
- Specific spices (cinnamon and turmeric)

We'll also avoid, or try to, the foods and beverages that can make it harder for your liver to do all of its important metabolic jobs.

- Limit, or better yet, avoid alcohol
- Stay away from deep-fried and high-fat foods
- Avoid smoked, cured, and heavily salted foods

I know it can be hard to part with some of the fatty "fun" foods you may be reaching for now, but trust me, you can do it for at least 15 days. Remember, on day 16, you can always go back to eating anything you'd like. If you don't feel better, look better, and have amazing energy—in short, if you don't feel like you're ready to blast off into your new life, then I'll eat my left shoe. Okay, that may sound extreme, but I KNOW this diet is meant for you. You're meant to lose the weight. You're meant to feel great. You're meant to be healthy. You're meant to eat this way.

Let me share one last thought to shepherd you into success: be honest with where you are, how you are doing, and whether you're truly taking care of yourself, and you will take off the pounds and get rid of the anchors that may be holding you down from blasting off into the body and life you want.

Up next: the four weight-loss weapons that will supercharge the plan to shed fat and pounds fastest. Read on because we're getting to the really good stuff soon, the delicious foods.

# 3

# SET . . .
# WHAT'S THE PLAN?

Now that you understand the truth about eating live, whole foods, as well as know the enormous health benefits that can result from specifically eating more plant foods, let's dive a little deeper into the exciting elements that form the core of the Blast Off Eating Plan.

This chapter is going to focus on four unique weight-loss tools. Each of these alone is a terrific asset in weight management, but taken together the results are astronomical. These health-inducing, fat-fighting food warriors will help you quickly jettison those unwanted pounds and unhealthy fat.

• Probiotics

• Prebiotics

• MCFAs (and other EFAs)

• Thermogenic Foods

If you're scratching your head, thinking you'll need a science degree to understand what some of these things are, don't worry. Really. I'll explain what these things are and why they're so great for you. But really all you have to do is reap the benefits—by enjoying the recipes. I don't believe in eating unpronounceable, processed foods or getting nutrition from pills and supplements. So why would I ask you to do so? Instead, as I've done in the rest of the book, I'll equip you with some pretty good reasons why you should be adding foods with these four fat fighters into your daily diet.

All the recipes and food choices you'll find here, what I call your Rocket Fuel, have been carefully selected to have one or more of these fat-fighting elements and only chosen for the plan after an extensive review of the most current research on nutrition and weight loss. I discovered some pretty exciting information through that reading— all of which will help you on your journey to the best type of melt down, a fat melt down. Before we jump into the diet, though, let's look a little more closely at our fuel sources and why we want to fill our tanks with them. Again, if you want to just jump to the diet, go ahead. It's your book. Your plan. I'm just arming you with as many reasons as possible to let me lead you on this journey to a gorgeously vibrant new you.

## ROCKET FUEL #1: PROBIOTICS—BELLY-FAT BLASTING 'BOTS?

You've likely heard of probiotics by now; yogurt commercials have been proclaiming their benefits for years, especially with regard to ensuring gut health. And you may have even heard of their promise in helping with type 2 diabetes and immune function. But did you know that scientists theorize that these little microbes may play a significant role in inducing or preventing obesity? Maybe even abdominal obesity— the dreaded belly fat?

But do you really understand what these critters are and what they do? It's really important to learn about these microflora because they're going to be your best friends from now on, particularly as they pertain to weight loss.

## PROBIOTICS 101

Researchers estimate that we have somewhere near 100 trillion microbes or microorganisms taking up space in or on our bodies. Many of these critters live in our guts; they are our unseen guests and use us, their unsuspecting hosts, to live. But before you get grossed out, keep reading. These bacteria are not all the same: some are good guests; some you want to kick out the back door, immediately.

We all know that some bacteria found in food can be deadly (*e. coli*, for example), but probiotics are a form of good-for-you bacteria, what I call, 'Bots. These bacteria are good for our digestive system, immune system, and our overall health, and they're good for fighting the bad guys. It is believed that some 70 percent of our immune system is localized, or established, in our intestinal tract. So keeping the balance of good guests to bad guests is key to keeping you healthy.

Also, when our digestive system is strong, it efficiently breaks down the foods we eat, helping us absorb and allocate nutrients to ensure we get the most out of our food. As I stated earlier, the stronger our digestion, the more efficient it is, and the more energy we have left over to be and to feel powerful.

A healthy gut also means waste is eliminated properly, rather than being stored in our belly and colon. Many of us hold onto 5 to 25 pounds of fecal matter in our bellies, depending on our diet and weight. Nasty! Imagine how much lighter we could be when we let that all go.

But good digestion and better assimilation of nutrients are not the only reasons I recommend probiotics on this plan. As I briefly mentioned earlier, there is some strong suggestion in the current scientific literature that obesity, and its recent rise, can't just be attributed to the imbalance of calories in versus calories out. Instead, researchers believe that the development of obesity (as well as Crohn's disease and type 1 diabetes) is influenced by other factors, such as the microflora in our gut. Translation: our metabolisms (and hence weight) are affected by the mix of bacteria in our gut, and probiotics are a promising tool in helping to regulate weight gain by providing more of the good guys, more of the 'Bots. In short, probiotics are believed to be a key weapon in fighting obesity, extracting more nutrition from your food, maintaining strong immune function, and protecting your body from chronic inflammation. I like to envision these bacterial beneficiaries as little 'Bots that are eating up belly fat and other unwanted extras in our bodies. They are in there doing battle for us.

So, what are good sources of probiotics? They can be found in pickled vegetables (like sauerkraut and kimchee), fermented drinks (like kombucha and kefir), and fermented foods like unpasteurized miso or apple cider vinegar—pretty much all fermented foods.

## What to Put in Your Tank

*Fermented soy products:*

    Miso

    Soy sauce

*Fermented drinks:*

    Kombucha

    Kefir

*Fermented vegetables:*

    Kimchee

    Pickles

    Sauerkraut

    Capers

*Other sources:*

    Apple cider vinegar, raw

    Nutritional yeast*

    Chocolate**

* Don't confuse this with brewer's yeast, which is used to brew beer. Nutritional yeast is yellow, flaky, and has a delicious cheesy flavor. It's an inactive yeast that is a great source of vitamin B12, especially good for vegans. You can find it in the bulk food section of your natural food store. In Australia and New Zealand, I hear that nutritional yeast is also known as "savory yeast flakes."

** Food researchers are experimenting with delivering probiotics through chocolates. And some studies to date have shown that two to three times more beneficial bacteria get delivered through this special chocolate as compared to dairy or yogurt. So I don't think it will hurt at all to try to eat a little dark chocolate with your probiotic foods—ideally raw chocolate and cacao powder, but any high-quality dark chocolate bar will work. It may just boost your weight loss.

### ☆ POWER PACKED: *Miso*

You now know that I love fermented foods for their probiotic effects and their flavor, and one of my favorites is fermented soybean paste or miso (also known as Chiang in China). A great source of protein (2 grams in 25 calories), as well as zinc, manganese, and copper, this condiment packs a great health punch. Always choose organic soy products to avoid GMOs (genetically modified organisms). Because organic soy is jam-packed with isoflavones and phytoestrogens, diets rich in this food have been associated with a number of health benefits, including the following:

- May help lower blood pressure in hypertensives
- May help reduce symptoms in peri-menopausal and menopausal women
- Helps to maintain bone health (soy is a good source of calcium)
- May help prevent prostate and breast cancers
- May help with atherosclerosis and cardiovascular risk (due to its isoflavones)
- Helps support immune function (due to its zinc content)

## ROCKET FUEL #2: PREBIOTICS—FEEDING THE 'BOTS

Prebiotics are a little trickier to understand; even scientists are still searching to define what exactly they are and how to classify them correctly. Here's my stab at it.

### PREBIOTICS 101

Prebiotics are substances in foods, often fibers or sugars, which promote the growth or activity of good bacteria in our bodies. They also improve the bioavailability of the nutrients in your foods—you get more nutrition from each bite you take. This bacteria is thought to create more SCFAs—short-chain fatty acids—which have been linked to positive health benefits for those suffering from Crohn's disease and high blood pressure, and possibly even preventing early stage colon cancer. Essential fatty acids (EFAs), particularly another class called medium-chain fatty acids (MCFAs), are another cool tool we'll discuss shortly.

Prebiotics are most commonly contained in foods with soluble fiber, but most any dietary fiber can have a prebiotic effect. There are no specific prebiotic foods, just foods that contain these fermentable buddies. Also, cooking destroys some of these fibers, so raw food sources are best. Just eat raw fruits and veggies!

Hard-to-pronounce terms warning: Oligofructose and inulin are two types of fructooligosaccharides (FOS) that have been well studied for their prebiotic effects. So our detox menus will include a diverse array of foods that contain them and other of these 'Bot helpers, including yummy stuff like garlic, asparagus, bananas, and honey. We want to eat more of them, so we've got more 'Bots on our side (well, in our insides) in the battle.

The plan doesn't forget synbiotics, either, which are foods that contain both probiotics and prebiotics. These provide even more health benefits. So we're going to stock up on them, too.

What else are these little instigators good for? Studies have linked prebiotics to improved cholesterol levels, cancer prevention, increased bone health, alleviating IBS discomfort and symptoms, and a slew more (and for the ladies, they may even help with PMS).

## What to Put in Your Tank

Asparagus

Bananas

Berries

Burdock

Chicory root

Flaxseed

Garlic, onion, leeks (Pile on any of the alliums.)

Greens: spinach, collards, chard, kale, mustard, dandelion

Honey

Jerusalem artichokes (Fun fact: these are different from artichokes; instead, they are root vegetables that come from a species of sunflower native to eastern North America. I love slicing them and using them as "chips" for my guacamole and hummus.)

Jicama

Tomatoes

## ROCKET FUEL #3: MCFAS (AND OTHER EFAS)—FATS THAT FIGHT FAT

I don't think any of us find it surprising that our parents were right when they told us to eat more fruits and vegetables; it's great advice for both overall health and a healthy weight.

But I do think many more of us are confused about eating fats. Are they healthy or not healthy? Which ones should you eat, and how much of them?

I'm not going to be the food police here and get involved in the fat wars, but I will try to clear up some of the confusion by saying that there are plenty of natural sources of healthy fats, and the ones we'll focus on in this plan will be rich in a group of fatty acids that are showing great promise in weight loss, MCFAs or medium-chain fatty acids. (You may also see these referred to as MCTs, too, which just stands for medium-chain triglycerides.)

What specifically makes them one of our key Rocket Fuels? Researchers believe they are potentially useful weapons in the fight against obesity by keeping body fat from accumulating and suppressing weight gain. Our bodies seem to "burn" these foods in such a way that we tend not to store their calories as fat. MCFAs basically bypass our storage containers (hips, belly, thighs, etc.) and are burned for energy instead. In short, they inhibit the depositing of fat within the body, which is good news for us! MCFAs seem to have better thermogenic qualities than other fatty acids; they increase "heat" in the body and energy expenditure (calorie burn). You'll also hear people refer to thermogenic foods as fat burners because of this added burn. (Don't worry, we've got a whole section coming next dedicated to foods that increase thermogenesis.) Bonus: MCFAs may make you feel satiated faster. It's a win-win.

But these fatty acids aren't the only ones we'll be utilizing for our Rocket Fuel. We'll also concentrate on MUFAs (monounsaturated fatty acids) and Omega 3s because of their weight loss benefits. Studies have shown that substituting MUFAs for saturated fats improves insulin levels and blood sugar—particularly helpful for type 2 diabetics. Omega 3s, as we mentioned earlier, are great for brain health, but did you know that they also stimulate the production of leptin, a hormone that helps regulate metabolism and weight? Ditching saturated fats and processed garbage and substituting foods that contain these fatty acids is taking a big step toward good health and a trim waist.

## What to Put in Your Tank

*MCFAs:*
- Coconut milk
- Coconut oil
- Palm kernel oil

*MUFAs:*
- Avocados
- Nuts
- Olive oil
- Seeds

*Omega 3s:*
- Flaxseed or flaxmeal
- Soybeans (cooked or sprouted, never raw)
- Walnuts

⭐ **POWER PACKED:** *Coconut Oil*

Coconut oil is not one of your Rocket Fuels for nothing. In addition to its promise in aiding weight loss, researchers have found that consuming it has these benefits:

- ■ May improve HDL cholesterol levels (in pre-menopausal women, in particular)
- ■ Good source of medium-chain fatty acids (about 55 percent to 65 percent of its content)
- ■ May have strong therapeutic benefit to those suffering from Crohn's disease (by reducing inflammation and decreasing the incidence of colitis)

■ Coconut oil is an antifungal, which means it's used to treat fungal infections. It kills yeast and candida, and it's also antibacterial. It attacks and kills viruses that have a fatty coating such as herpes, HIV, hepatitis C, flu, and mononucleosis.

Now, don't go running off thinking that a coconut candy bar is the best source for this. Look closer to the ground or toward the sky for fresh coconuts on the ground or in a palm tree. Or, just use a high-quality unrefined and unbleached coconut oil, aka coconut butter, to access healthy MCFA's.

 ## ROCKET FUEL #4: THERMOGENIC FOODS

If you're like most people, you are super busy. Full days, full nights, full weeks, full weekends, and full months. You're running through your life at hyper speed, and you have way too much on your to-do list. You likely find yourself multitasking, even when you'd rather be slowing down and living life at a more manageable speed. Why not put your food to work for you, so there's one area of your life where you don't have to overdo it? Let it multitask for you, providing multiple benefits in every bite. And that's what you'll get from this next group of Rocket Fuels. Hardworking foods with health and fat-burning powers. We know the drill: If you burn more calories, you should lose more weight. But how about this one: *Eat the right foods, and they will actually accelerate your metabolism.* You can eat them for great health and for their calorie burn.

Thermogenesis is a fancy word for fat-burning foods. They are metabolically active, functional foods (have a positive effect on health) that can aid in weight loss. These foods, just by being their own fabulous selves, actually increase the number of calories you expend, and you don't have to do anything but sit back and enjoy this benefit.

## ⭐ POWER PACKED: *Chilies*

The capsaicin in chile peppers is what gives them the heat they are known for bringing to any food party in your mouth. But did you know that it and the peppers also:

■ May help fight prostate cancer (by stopping the cells from replicating themselves)

■ Paradoxically, can help with the burn you feel with indigestion and may help prevent stomach ulcers (might be due to making the environment not too friendly to unfriendly bacteria)

■ Can help temporarily manage localized pain (when topically applied)

■ May reduce inflammation, help reduce cholesterol and triglycerides, lower the risk of type 2 diabetes, and improve immunity

■ Help fight colds (by clearing out congestion in your lungs and nasal passages)

Bring on the burn!

I'm sure you've by now heard we should all drink more green tea. It's the ultimate multitasker. But did you know it is one of the best fat-burning foods, especially for tackling belly fat? Green tea is high in a type of flavanol called catechins, specifically one called EGCG (hard-to-pronounce word alert: epigallocatechin gallate). Scientists have found that foods containing catechins produce more abdominal fat loss.

## ⭐ POWER PACKED: *Green Tea*

If you do just a quick search of PubMed (a great research site provided by the National Institutes of Health, www.ncbi.nlm.nih.gov/pubmed), you'll find well over 100 articles on green tea alone. Here's what I found that you should know.

Habitual consumption of green tea:

- Shows promise in the treatment of arthritis (because of its EGCG)
- Provides a significant genoprotective effect (translation: it enhances DNA repair)
- May protect against breast, prostate, colorectal, and lung cancers
- Shows promise for weight management, decreasing cardiovascular risk factors, and glucose control for type 2 diabetics
- Is associated with a decrease in all-cause mortality

So drink up. What have you got to lose (besides unwanted extra fat)?

Green tea is the best source of catechins, but I've also included foods below that have much smaller amounts of them, with the thought that the sum is greater than the parts. Or to put it more simply: it can't hurt if weight loss is your goal to pile on foods that just might help you increase your calorie burn, especially those that have other great health benefits to boot.

I've added other great spices, foods, and drinks that are also great fat burners. You have likely heard that caffeine is one, but did you know the temperature of the water you drink could affect fat burn? Or that cayenne pepper can do more than heat up your mouth?

Read on and tank up.

## What to Put in Your Tank

Black pepper

Caffeine

Calcium-rich* foods such as blackstrap molasses; collard, mustard, and turnip greens; sesame seeds; spinach

Cayenne

Grapefruit

Ginger

Green tea**

Ice water

Lean protein like buckwheat groats, brown rice protein powder, and seeds

Turmeric

Vitamin D-rich* mushrooms, including shiitake mushrooms

*Researchers found that a higher calcium and vitamin D intake at the morning meal significantly increased diet-induced thermogenesis over the span of the next two meals, as well.

**Apples, blackberries, strawberries, nuts, avocados, plums, onions, and raspberries all have EGCGs, too, but in very small amounts. It's unknown whether the trace amounts of catechins in these foods have a true thermogenic effect, but as I said earlier, it can't hurt to eat these great foods for their other health benefits alone.

I hope you're now revved up and ready to go. If you join me on this journey, together we'll put all the fuel in your body it needs to have it (and you) performing at its prime, while shedding weight painlessly. I can't wait for you to taste just how great my recipes are.

Next up is a quick peek at the 15-day plan and tips for stocking your refrigerator and counters with what you'll need to get started. We've gotten ready and set; now it's time to go!

# GO! THE DIET BASICS

Now we get to the really fun part: eating! Well, we're almost there. This chapter reviews the basic diet plan and how to follow it for best success, as well as providing tips on getting started so your kitchen is stocked and you're able to go!

First we'll take a quick walk through the next 15 days of your life and how to live the plan in a way that best fits your personality, needs, and lifestyle. No matter where you're starting, I'll arm you with the tools you'll need to make it simple and seamless. Then we'll head to the supermarket to stock up on what you need. But first, let's look at what the next two weeks plus are going to bring to your plate.

## THE RAW FOOD DETOX DIET: PLAN BASICS

There are three phases to this 15-day plan, and they focus on slightly different goals. Overall, the plan has but one major purpose: to help you blast off the fat and the pounds, while shooting your health into the stratosphere. Phase 1, Shake It Up, is a cleansing phase and is short, just three days, which is long enough to give you a clean engine with which to begin your new journey. Phase 2, Melt Down, will launch you through the rest of the week by focusing on probiotics, prebiotics, and MCFAs as major sources of your fuel for major fat melt down. Phase 3, Blast Off, uses our Rocket Fuel groups with a laser focus on thermogenic fat-blasting ingredients in each and every meal and recipe. It's designed to synergistically knock down whatever remaining barriers stand in the way of a lean, trim you.

There's nothing to fear here; just jump in and make yourself comfortable. It's all good. Everyone has his or her own speed of weight loss, as well as comfort level with what I'm suggesting you eat. Go at your own speed. The plan works best when followed exactly as I've written it, but if you find that you just don't want to do it the way I've crafted it, then start with any of the phases, even mix and match them: you'll still get great benefits. But do try it my way, first. Okay?

Here's a quick look at the basics of the plan.

## PHASE 1—SHAKE IT UP (DAYS 1–3)

As I've just stated, the first three days on this plan are meant to be a detox. The foods will begin to clear out the fat in your body where toxins are stored and provide you and your body with a clean slate from which to work the plan, as well as a quick jumpstart to weight loss. Losing weight this quickly acts as a great impetus for sticking with the rest of the plan. Nothing is more motivating than success! You'll be drinking lots of healthy shakes and soups that are filled with some of my favorite health-promoting foods from our four Rocket Fuel categories. Yet this phase will have a special focus on those ingredients that have mega cleaning and scrubbing power to get you squeaky clean. Think anti-inflammatory and alkaline foods. The menus and meals during this stage will often include pineapple, ginger, lemon, coconut oil, cinnamon, and cayenne—cleansing foods that are rich with enzymes, nutrients, and phytochemicals that will help you power launch into the next stage.

### ☆ Drink Up

I recommend drinking at least eight 8-ounce glasses of water a day. Personally, I drink 3 to 4 liters—about 1 gallon—daily. Slicing cucumbers into your water is delicious, but squeezing lemon or lime juice into your water acts as a debriding agent that will keep your engines squeaky clean!

## PHASE 2—MELT DOWN (DAYS 4–7)

Each phase in the plan is additive, in that we carry over some of the great foods used in the prior phase and then add even more Rocket Fuels as we travel along on our weight-loss journey. Here, we'll add in prebiotic and probiotic foods, so we can let the 'Bots come in and eat up the belly and other fat you want to get rid of. We also add in more MCFAs, the healthy fats that actually help us melt fat away, so these Rocket Fuels can work to melt off fat, so you don't have to!

In Phase 2, we will shift from a purely liquid diet to getting lean and green by adding in a salad for lunch, with an option to continue enjoying your shake as your morning snack. You can also substitute it out for a solid meal, if you're feeling the need to chew on something.

### Tailor the Plan to Your Needs

If you have more than 10 to 15 pounds to lose, then you might choose to repeat Phases 1 and 2 in sequence a couple times to turbocharge your Melt Down before moving on to Phase 3. You can also choose to repeat Phases 2 and 3 in sequence for as long as you need to get to your goal weight. This is your diet, and you can pick and choose the phases as they suit you. But don't keep repeating Phase 1 on its own; I don't advocate that length of detox. It's too hard on the body long-term.

## PHASE 3—BLAST OFF (DAYS 8–15)

For days 8 through 15, we'll focus on combining everything we've learned up to that point to get as much of a synergistic effect as possible to help you reach your end goal and prep you for continuing your health journey. We'll incorporate more solid foods for dinner, too, while still drinking a daily, nutrient rich, fat-blasting, 'Bot-containing shake or smoothie. Every meal in this phase uses all four Rocket Fuels to help you jettison the remaining pounds. I'll get to show off my tasty wraps, soups, meals, even desserts and sweet treats. All are part of this phase of your trip.

## SETTING UP YOUR KITCHEN FOR THE 15-DAY DETOX

You're raring to go now. But how do you get started? Everything starts for me in the kitchen. First up, the tools you'll need.

### KITCHEN ESSENTIALS

We're all busy juggling a gazillion things in our day, so having the right tools in your kitchen will make food prep super easy and quick. Setting up your kitchen at home, or even your office, to make fresh, raw food recipes is simple. Having the right tools makes food prep enjoyable and fun! The thing is, the tools you'll need for this diet are the same tools you'd find in any kitchen. My two basics are a blender and a food processor.

### High-Speed Blender

A blender is used on this plan to whip up yummy liquid concoctions, like shakes, soups, sauces, and dressings. Some blenders come with or have as an option a second "dry" container that can be used to grind nuts and seeds into powder form, or what's called meal. I avoid using my wet blender container to grind these foods because I don't want to dull the blades. A coffee grinder works great for grinding smaller quantities of nuts and small seeds like flax or chia, for example.

I always recommend saving up your pennies to buy one really good high-speed blender. There are many brands to choose from including Vitamix, Waring, and BlendTec. These blenders cost as much as $400 to $500, but they're well worth it if you can afford them. Some might argue that you can't put a price on health, and I'd be one of them. But you have to look to what your pocketbook can and can't do. Realize these tools will last a LONG time. I've used my blenders to make food for thousands of people in my commercial kitchen, and they're still going strong. Besides lasting a lifetime, these high-speed blenders pulverize ingredients to give you a smooth, fluffy texture.

It's okay if you're still saving up for a high-speed blender. It could take a while. So, in the meantime, any blender will work just fine. Keep in mind that your mixture may not come out as smooth, and chunks of nuts could remain in the mix. If this bothers you, I recommend you grind down nuts and seeds into a powder first to ease the load on your blender.

 I also have a smaller blender with 1-, 2-, and 3-cup containers that I like to use when making batches that are too small for a high-speed blender container (volumes less than 1½ to 2 cups). My personal blender comes with a grinder attachment, too, which I use as my grinder. Smaller blenders are nice to have and are great for stuffing into your suitcase when you travel. If you don't have one, you can always double or triple smaller batches to create more volume to blend in your larger, high-speed blender. That means even less time for you to "not-cook" these meals.

### Food Processor

A food processor chops dry and low-moisture ingredients like nuts, larger seeds (like sunflower), and vegetables. They cost about $50 to $100. An alternative to food processing is old-school chopping by hand, which will take much longer than just turning on a switch to let the machine do it for you in a few seconds. Having a food processor will make it so much simpler and faster to whip up some of the recipes in Phase 3 of the plan.

### Notebook

I always keep a notebook and pens and pencils in my kitchen for taking notes and writing down all my favorite recipes. I pretty much write down everything I make, and I have a rating system for tagging the recipes that I really liked. Having a bunch of tried and true recipes on hand makes it easy to put together a quick meal at the last minute, too. Give it a try.

## NICE-TO-HAVES, NOT MUST-HAVES

### Spiralizer

I have noodle recipes that are fun to make using a spiralizer, also known as a spiral cutter or Saladacco, which is used to slice vegetables into long strips, shaped much like angel hair pasta. You can always slice veggies by hand into flat fettuccine noodle shapes if you don't have a spiralizer. One model of spiralizer comes in at about $25 to $35 and is available online at www.GoSuperLife.com.

### Vegetable Peeler

A vegetable peeler will help you peel a thin layer of skin off fruits and vegetables. It can also be used to slice vegetables into thin strips for vegetable noodles.

### Vegetable Juicer

I opted not to require a juicer for this book, though I do have several in my kitchen. I make green vegetable juices almost daily and drink about a pint of green juice to ensure I get a ton of vitamins, minerals, enzymes, and nourishment into my body each day. Green juice is my equivalent to taking a daily multivitamin. Things I like to juice include cabbage, kale, chard, lemons, cucumber, jalapeño, cilantro, parsley, and celery. Almost immediately, I can see my skin glow with radiant health and vitality.

If you have a juicer, definitely use it and add a green juice daily to this program if you'd like. You'll feel amazing, plus, it shows up in your skin, hair, nails, and kicks up your overall vitality.

Vitality = Beauty!

### Mason Jars

I save all my glass jars and reuse them to store my nuts, seeds, dried fruits, hemp protein powder, flax meal, dried herbs, and spices. Glass jars are great for storing shakes, sauces, and dressings, too. Make sure you have a selection of different-sized jars on hand for storing ingredients and also for carrying shakes and food with you when you're on the go.

### Citrus Juicer

This is nice to have, especially when you need to juice a lot of lemons for lemonade. But it's pretty simple to just squeeze limes and lemons by hand, too.

## Knives

Obtain several knives of various sizes. I prefer ceramic knives because they don't oxidize cut veggies and fruits like metal does, and mine don't seem to ever need sharpening. Ceramic knives are available online at www.GoSuperLife.com.

## Whisk

A whisk is fun to have, but you can always use a spoon or fork to mix and beat liquids together.

## Mixing bowls

Gather mixing bowls of various sizes, from small to large. Glass is always best, but it's heavy. The bowls I use most frequently at home are stainless steel, from my commercial kitchen, because they're rugged and light.

## Dehydrator

This is a tool you don't need for our 15-day program, but you may want to consider acquiring one later for making healthy treats and snacks. A dehydrator is used to dry food at low temperatures and simulates sun-drying. In the hotter months, especially in the desert, you can dehydrate simply by placing food on a baking tray in the sun. But for those of us who don't have that luxury, a dehydrator extracts moisture from whatever's put inside.

There are many models of dehydrators on the market to choose from. My favorite is still the nine-tray Excalibur with built-in timer. I recommend purchasing the reusable nonstick Paraflexx liners, too.

Once you have a dehydrator, you can make kale chips, which have become so popular. Folks try making them in the oven, but often they'll burn them because even on low, the oven's temp is too high. I have the most delicious Cheddar-Kale Chip recipe in *Ani's Raw Food Essentials*, page 110. I like to think I invented kale chips when I had a bunch of dressed Kale Salad left over from a catering gig. Rather than tossing it out or feeding it to Kanga, my pooch, I put the salad into my dehydrator for about four hours. I was thrilled with the end product! Today, I make about three batches of kale chips a week to snack on. They travel amazingly well, even when biking all day long. You can't beat chips that are salad! Yummy.

## ⭐ Picking Your Produce

Choose local, seasonal, and organic food whenever possible. Seasonal food is at its peak in both flavor and nutrient value, so you get more for your money. Plus, local food travels less and is handled less, which lower the chances of contamination by some dangerous food-borne illness. I choose organic when available to avoid eating poisonous herbicides, pesticides, "natural" flavors, colors, and preservatives.

I love shopping at farmers' markets, which go year round here in Los Angeles. Produce arrives super fresh, usually just picked a few hours earlier. You'll definitely notice how much longer this food lasts. And less spoilage = less money wasted. The market has become my community, and I look forward to visiting with the farmers each week.

Buying directly from individual farmers means you're buying in bulk, avoiding environmentally unfriendly packaging, and treading lighter on our planet. Plus, all the money you spend goes directly to the farmer, rather than to packaging, manufacturing, distributing, storing, and advertising.

Biodiverse organic farming produces more food for farmers. It means the farm is not mono-cropped to grow only one type of food. Instead, there's an entire ecosystem that thrives in a biodiverse garden or farm.

Here's a tip for shopping at grocery stores. Grab weekly circulars from as many different stores as you can and note weekly sale items that are priced low to bring you into the store. If you've got the time, it's worth shopping at various stores to save money by buying these sale items.

## 15-DAY RAW FOOD PANTRY + FRIDGE

Keeping your kitchen stocked with a few basic ingredients will help make it easy to whip up a healthy snack or meal at a moment's notice. Here's a high-level view of some items I always keep in my kitchen. I provide it here so you can get an idea of how you can set the stage for success for yourself, even when you're not doing the 15-Day plan. Specific shopping lists for each phase of the diet follow as well.

## Nuts, seeds, herbs, spices, superfoods, and oils

I always have several varieties of nuts and seeds stored in glass jars in my pantry including walnuts, almonds, cashews, sunflower seeds, pumpkin seeds, black and tan sesame seeds, and chia seeds. I also keep dry herbs and spices in glass jars including oregano, thyme, dill, and chipotle powder. Superfoods I keep on hand include sea vegetables like nori, dulse, arame, wakame; powders like camu camu, maca, matcha, green tea, dehydrated barley grass, alfalfa grass, wheatgrass, and blue green algae like spirulina and chlorella; cacao powder and nibs; and dried super fruits like goji berries and golden berries. I keep various oils around including hemp, olive, flax, coconut, sesame, and sacha inchi. Most of these oils are easily found at natural food stores. If you're new to sacha inchi, it has been used by indigenous people of the Peruvian Amazon for thousands of years, and is a great source of Omega 3s. Check out the sidebar at the end of this chapter if you're stumped by any of the other staple ingredients I commonly use. They may sound unusual, but they rock!

## Fruits, vegetables, nut butters, and unpasteurized miso

I store fresh produce in the refrigerator, and I buy whatever looks good at the market. I always keep longer-lasting staples like lemons, limes, cabbage, onion, garlic, jalapeño, and celery on hand because I use them so frequently, and they last at least a couple of weeks when stored in airtight containers.

## STOW AWAYS: HOW TO STORE FOOD SMARTLY AND SAFELY

To avoid mold and decay in your fridge, keep fruits and vegetables stored separately because they both give off different gasses that can accelerate deterioration. Store similar items together, like apples with apples, and lettuce with lettuce. For leftovers, store them in airtight, leak-proof, clear containers so you can always see what's inside. Glass jars work great. And keep items with shorter shelf lives toward the front of your fridge; items that will last longer should be placed in the back. As you gobble up the stuff in front, the stuff in back moves forward to be used next. Always store animal products (if using), like meats, on the bottom shelf of the fridge on a dish to catch their juices and keep food-borne bacteria contained.

# GO SHOPPING: THE DETOX SHOPPING LIST

I've compiled shopping lists for each of the three phases of this plan to make it easy for you to quickly jump right into your raw food eating plan. These shopping lists are designed so that you can easily follow the phases in order, from 1 to 3. I've also broken out staple ingredients you should always keep on hand in your kitchen to make food prep fast and simple. I'll start first with the staples with which to stock your kitchen, then we'll move to the fresh ingredients that are specific to each phase. Be forewarned that the list of staples may be a long one. They are meant to hold you over throughout the plan, so please don't be intimidated by the list. Some of these ingredients may be new to you, but again, please try them because you might love them! Most can be found at www.GoSuperLife.com if you can't find them at your natural food store.

## STAPLES (FOR ALL THREE PHASES)

### Nuts and seeds (always raw and unsalted)

Almonds, 1½ lbs

Cashews, 1 lb

Dry coconut, 4 oz (unsweetened, shredded)

Flax seeds, 4 oz

Pecans, ½ lb

Pistachios, ½ lb

Pumpkin seeds, 4 oz

Sesame seeds, small bag or jar (tan or black)

Sunflower seeds, ½ lb

Walnuts, 1 lb

Hemp protein powder, if using, 1 lb

Brown rice protein powder if using, 1 kg (2.2 lbs)
  (bio-fermented, sprouted)

# ☆ POWER PACKED: *Walnuts*

Many folks have feared eating nuts because of their high fat and calorie content, but these little guys are definitely friends not foes in both the battle of the bulge and in giving your body what it needs for optimal health. Go nuts for these nuts (unless you're allergic to them; if that's the case, reach for the flaxseed instead), and you'll reap the following benefits:

■ Natural chemoprevention: researchers believe the high anti-oxidant content in nuts may be responsible for their potentially potent chemopreventive (protect against the development of cancer) action.

■ Better heart health: high intakes of walnuts are associated with cardiovascular improvements such as lower cholesterol and less arterial stiffness. A walnut-rich diet may reduce cardiovascular risk in type 2 diabetics, as well.

■ Help with PCOS (polycystic ovary syndrome): a recent study at UC Davis showed that eating walnuts (or almonds) exuded a beneficial effect on both lipids (blood fats) and androgens for those suffering from this endocrine disorder.

■ Limit belly fat: walnut and flaxseed may be particularly helpful with central obesity (belly fat) in those with the metabolic syndrome.

And if you're still worried about fat and calories, grab some pistachios: they aren't, as of yet, known to pack the same health punch of walnuts, but they are a great source of protein and a pretty "lean" nut.

## Dried Fruits

Raisins, 1 lb (unsulfured)
Medjool dates, 1 lb

## Oils

Coconut oil, 16 oz jar (extra virgin, unheated, raw, unbleached)
Olive oil, small bottle, about 8 oz or 250 ml (extra virgin, cold pressed)
Sesame oil, small bottle, about 8 oz or 250 ml (toasted)
Hemp oil, if using, small bottle, about 8 oz or 250 ml
Flax oil, if using, small bottle, about 8 oz or 250 ml

## Condiments

Apple cider vinegar, small bottle, or 32 oz (unfiltered, raw)
Black olives, 1/4 cup (fresh, not canned)
Cacao nibs, small bag, about 4 oz (raw, unheated)
Cacao powder, or cocoa powder, small bag, about 4 oz
Miso paste, 16 oz (unpasteurized, any color)
Nama shoyu (raw soy sauce), or Tamari (gluten-free), small bottle, about 8 oz or 250 ml
Sauerkraut, jar, about 12 oz (raw, unpasteurized, refrigerated)
Capers, small jar, about 7 oz

## Dried spices and herbs

Black pepper, powder, small bag or jar, or peppercorns with grinder, about 1.2 oz
Cayenne, powder, small bag, 1.2 oz
Chipotle, powder, small bag, 1.2 oz
Cinnamon, small bottle, 1.8 oz
Cumin seeds, small bag, about 1.2 oz
Curry, powder, small bag, 1.2 oz
Dill, dry, small bag, about 1.2 oz
Sea salt, small bag, 1.2 oz
Turmeric, small bag, 1.2 oz
Oregano, small bag, 1.2 oz
Rosemary, small bag, 1.2 oz
Thyme, small bag, 1.2 oz

Basil, small bag, 1.2 oz

Nutritional yeast, 1 cup

Vanilla flavor or extract, 1 bottle, 4 fl oz,
   or 4 whole beans (alcohol free)

## Green tea

Matcha powder, small bottle, 2.8 oz, or box of tea bags
   (16 count or more)

## Sweeteners

Stevia powder, 1.5 oz (whole leaf green)

Syrups, one or more, small bottle each, if using, about 8 oz: agave,
   maple (grade B), brown rice, palm nectar, raw honey

## Produce

Celery, 1 bunch

Garlic, 1 bulb

Ginger, ¼ cup (fresh)

Jalapeños, 2 whole

Lemons, 8 whole

Limes, 4 whole

## Sea vegetables

Nori sheets, small pack, 10 sheets (raw)

Wakame or arame, ½ cup dry

## Super Power Pack (bonus superfoods), optional

Kelp noodles, 1 bag

Bee pollen, small bag

Dulse, small bag (flakes or whole)

Maca, 2 tablespoons (powder)

Spirulina, small bottle, 5 oz (powder)

Chlorella, small bottle, 5 oz (powder)

Chlorella, tablets, small bag, if using, to snack on

Wheatgrass, small bottle, 5 oz or bag, 8 oz (dehydrated powder)

Kombucha or nondairy water or coconut Kefir, six bottles or more to
   enjoy throughout the program

## PHASE 1: SHAKE IT UP RECIPE INGREDIENTS

### Fruit

Blueberries, 1 cup (fresh or frozen)

Strawberries, 1 cup (fresh or frozen)

Pineapple, 2 cups (fresh or frozen)

Avocados, 4 whole

Tomatoes, 4 medium

Apple, any type, 1 whole

Pear, 1 whole

### Vegetables

Kale, any type, 2 to 3 big leaves, or 1 small head

Ginger, ¼ cup (fresh)

Baby bok choy, or regular, 1 cup, about 2 large leaves, or 1 small
    bunch or head

Cucumbers, 2 whole

Jalapeño, 1 whole

Romaine, about 2 to 3 large leaves, or 1 small head

Spinach, 1 cup, or 1 small bunch, or a small pre-washed bag

### Herbs and spices

Cilantro, 1 tablespoon, or 1 small bunch (fresh)

Oregano, 1 teaspoon, or 1 small bunch (fresh)

Rosemary, 1 teaspoon, or 1 small bunch (fresh)

Thyme, 1 teaspoon, or 1 small bunch (fresh)

## PHASE 2: MELT DOWN RECIPE INGREDIENTS

### Fruits

Apples, 2 whole (any type)

Avocados, 4 whole

Bananas, 3 whole

Blueberries, 1½ cups, about 1 pint (fresh)

Grapefruit, 2 whole

Mango, 2 cups, about 2 whole (fresh or frozen)

Pineapple, 3½ cups fresh ideally, or frozen

Pomegranate seeds, ½ cup, 1 whole

Strawberries, 1 cup (fresh or frozen)

Tomatoes, 4 medium

## Vegetables

Broccoli, ½ cup

Cabbage, napa, 2 cups, about ½ head

Carrot, 1 whole

Corn, 1 ear (fresh)

Cucumbers, 2 medium

Kale, 1 large leaf, or 1 small bunch or head

Mesclun salad mix, 5 cups

Radishes, 3 whole

Spinach, 3 cups, or 1 pre-washed bag, or 1 bunch

Red leaf lettuce, 3 to 4 leaves, or 1 small head

Romaine, 1½ cups, about 6 leaves, or 1 small head

Red bell pepper, 1 medium

Sprouts, any type, 1 cup

## Herbs and spices

Basil, 2 tablespoons, or 1 small bunch (fresh)

Cilantro, 1 tablespoon, or 1 small bunch

Dill, 2 tablespoons, or 1 small bunch (fresh)

Mint, ¼ cup, lightly packed, or 1 to 2 bunches (fresh)

## PHASE 3: BLAST OFF RECIPE INGREDIENTS

## Fruits

Avocados, 7 medium

Banana, 1 whole

Blueberries, fresh 2½ cups, or fresh ½ cup + frozen 2 cups

Grapefruit, 3 whole

Oranges, 2 whole

Peaches, 2 whole

Pears, 2 whole (any type)

Pineapple, 1¼ cups, about ½ whole (frozen or fresh)

Strawberries, fresh, 4½ cups, or frozen, 2 cups + fresh, 2½ cups
Watermelon, 1 cup (fresh)

## Vegetables

Cabbage, 1 small head (any type)
Carrots, 4 medium
Collard greens, 3 large leaves, or 1 small bunch
Cucumber, 8 medium
Fennel, 2 cups, or 1 large bulb
Jicama, 1 medium
Mushrooms: shiitake, crimini, or portabella, 2 cups
Red bell peppers, 3 medium
Romaine, 1 head
Red leaf lettuce, ½ head
Scallions, 1 bunch
Sprouts, 2½ cups
Tomatoes, 2 cups (cherry)
Tomatoes, 4 medium
Zucchini, 3 medium

## Herbs and spices

Basil, 1½ cups, lightly packed, 1 to 2 large bunches (fresh)
Cilantro, ⅔ cup, 1 large bunch (fresh)
Dill, 1 tablespoon, 1 small bunch (fresh)
Mint, 1 tablespoon, 1 small bunch
Oregano, 2 tablespoons, 1 small bunch (fresh)
Rosemary, 1 teaspoon, 1 small bunch (fresh)

Now just how do you use all these yummy fresh foods? Flip to Chapter 5 and see how all of these come together to create the delicious treats you'll be putting on your plate for the next 15 days.

## ⭐ Detox Foods
## You May Have Never Heard of or Used

### Alfalfa grass juice powder

I like dehydrated grass powders because I can have a mineral-rich green juice without a juicer, which is particularly useful when traveling. The powders can be added to a glass of water or any shake. Alfalfa grass, like barley grass and wheatgrass, is a potent source of antioxidants and phytochemicals. Alfalfa grass is used in traditional Chinese and Ayurvedic medicine to treat poor digestion, arthritis, kidney stones, and other digestive issues. It has a sweet, mild flavor that makes adding it to shakes simple, and it is super alkalizing, shifting our pH levels from acidic to more alkaline and boosting our immune systems.

### Barley grass juice powder

Barley grass powder is a super food that has 22 times the iron found in spinach, four times the calcium of dairy milk, and as much protein per ounce as a steak. It helps with just about everything from anti-aging to weight loss. Its powder form has a mild, sweet flavor, which makes it easy to mix these greens into your water, shake, or smoothie.

### Brown rice protein powder

If you've ever had a smoothie at a health food bar, it was likely made with whey protein or milk protein. But here we're going to focus on a great nonallergenic source: brown rice. Rice protein has been shown to be highly digestible and is a great choice for those who have known milk allergies or who object to animal proteins. Some people feel brown rice protein powder has a chalky texture, but I don't mind it. Brown rice protein powder helps us increase our protein intake, and because protein has a thermic effect, to speed up fat burning.

### Buckwheat groats

Buckwheat groats are the hulled seeds of the buckwheat plant. These soft white seeds have a mild flavor. Buckwheat is gluten free, so it is a suitable substitute for those who are wheat or grain sensitive. This high-quality protein is a good source of manganese, magnesium, and fiber. I like to soak and sprout the groats in triple the amount of filtered water overnight (i.e., 1 cup groats in 3 cups water) and then dehydrate them to make "crispies" that I use to top salads and soups, sprinkle into wraps, and add crunch to desserts.

### Cacao nibs and powder

Cacao is simply the fruit you know as chocolate. You can get it as beans, in little nibs of the bean, and in powdered form. Within the cacao pod are the seeds known as cacao beans. The beans look somewhat like coffee beans and break apart into cacao nibs. Cacao beans and nibs contain about 40 percent fat, which is extracted as cocoa butter. The remaining powder is known as cacao powder. Cacao is a terrific source of sulfur and magnesium, and it's believed that certain enzyme inhibitors in raw cacao can diminish your appetite, which is great for a detox! Look for unroasted and unsweetened cacao beans and nibs.

### Camu Camu

Camu Camu is a plant found along rivers and lakes in Peru, Brazil, and Venezuela that produces a grape-sized, red and purple berry containing the highest recorded source of vitamin C on the planet— about 30 times that of oranges and lemons. The berries of the Camu Camu plant are juiced after harvest and then freeze dried. They can be blended into juices and smoothies, where its dried pink powder adds a fruity, semi-sweet, acidic flavor.

### Chlorella

Chlorella is an algae found in fresh water. It is believed to boost immunity, help detox heavy metals, and even eliminate constipation and body odor. Chlorella contains mostly protein, vitamins like E, B, and C, as well as minerals like zinc and iron. It comes in a dried pow- der, and this powder is also pressed into tablets. I enjoy snacking on the tablets throughout my day because I love the flavor. People say it tastes like seaweed and green tea.

### Goji berries

Gojis are a delicious, sweet, bright orange-red berry, about the same size as a raisin; they are also known as wolfberry. They come from a shrub native to China and have been eaten for centuries to increase longevity. Some research suggests that Gojis' antioxidants and vitamins help boost brain health, while also protecting against Alzheimer's.

### Golden berries

Originally from the Andes, golden berries are sweet and tart and are a little larger than a raisin. They contain tiny seeds that give these berries a slight crunchy texture. They are high in phosphorous, calcium, B vitamins, as well as vitamins A and C; and they are also high in protein. Enjoy them as you would any berry or raisins, in trail mix, cereals, and cookies and salads.

### Hemp protein powder

Though this food might be new to you, hemp is a crop that has been cultivated in this country since colonial times. George Washington and Thomas Jefferson even farmed it! It has been and continues to be used in many household products, including clothes and foods. The powder I recommend you use on this plan is created by cold pressing the hemp seed to remove its oil, leaving behind one heck of a nutrient profile: about 45 percent protein, 43 percent fiber, and 9 percent beneficial fats.

### Maca

Maca is a Puruvian superfood from the Andes, which is considered an adaptogen because it rebuilds weak immune systems, remineralizes poorly nourished bodies, and increases energy and endurance. It can be found in powder form at your natural food store and at www.GoSuperLife.com.

### Matcha

Matcha is a finely milled green tea that is packed with antioxidants and has been reported to boost metabolism, enhance mood, lower cholesterol, and help balance blood sugar. Green tea leaves, whose veins and stems have been removed, are ground into a powder. One cup of matcha is believed to be equal to 100 cups of other green teas in terms of nutritional value and antioxidant levels. I love the flavor of green tea, and this powder is easy to add to shakes and smoothies for added anti-aging, antioxidant, and fat-burning boosts.

### Sacha inchi

This Peruvian plant grows small nuts that are rich in oil that is both cholesterol-free and Omega 3-rich. It's a tasty source of vitamins A and E and is high in protein, rich in essential and nonessential amino acids, and has a strong nutty flavor similar to hemp oil. Sacha inchi can be used as you would use any oil, in dressings, sauces, and soups, or just drizzled onto your recipe before serving. Because it has a such a strong flavor, you may want to use it sparingly or mix it with a milder oil like olive oil.

### Spirulina

Spirulina is a microscopic blue-green algae that can be found at natural food stores as flakes, powder, and pressed tablets. It tastes like seaweed and has a strong ocean aroma. Spirulina contains high amounts of protein, essential amino acids, essential fatty acids, vitamins, and minerals. As with chlorella, spirulina boosts the immune system, aids in digestion, and helps our bodies become more alkaline (which is a good thing).

# PART 2

# RAW FOOD DETOX: THE 15-DAY COUNTDOWN

# 5

# DETOX MENUS
# AND DIET PLAN

Yum. That's all I have to say here. And it's what you'll be saying, too, when you dive into the delicious foods we'll prepare together during all three phases.

You have 15 days of meal plans, laid out for you here. From shakes to soups, salads, wraps, rolls, noodles, and even desserts. Each meal will be replete with healthy fats and proteins, as well as tons of fresh whole foods, fruits, and vegetables. And best of all, remember how I told you this was easy? These take minimal time to prepare because they are minimally processed foods. You'll have ample time to enjoy eating them, as well as enjoy whatever else you love to do . . . or have to do. Plus, in creating this plan, my focus as a chef has been on giving you delicious, nutritious, satisfying recipes so you won't feel tortured or deprived.

In this chapter, I share the menus for each day with the titles of the recipes you will be enjoying. This makes following the program super simple. I also offer motivational tips at the beginning of each day to keep this fun. At the end of each day, you can write notes about any challenges you encountered, as well as how you feel. Pretty much all the folks who have tested this program say they feel lighter, tighter, more energetic, find their focus to be clearer, and feel vibrant. But this is your space; use it to dig into whatever issue you find yourself facing during the day.

When we start on a new path there are unique obstacles and hills and valleys that we encounter; use the space on each day's page to write down yours. You'll be able to come back to read what you've written and remind yourself how far you've come, and it will help keep you motivated too. If you don't want to write in the book, buy a notebook and dedicate it to your health journey; use your computer, etc. I've also included some sample journaling pages at the back of the book—you can write there or photocopy them to create your own journal—whatever you like.

## 🖉 Why Do This?

Before you start the detox, I want you to write down, below or in a separate notebook or at the back of this book, your motivation for picking up this book and for wanting to lose weight. Come back to visit your notes whenever you need to motivate yourself and remember why you're doing this in the first place:

I want to lose weight because . . .

_____

_____

I need to lose weight because . . .

_____

_____

I will allow myself to change and become healthier because . . .

_____

_____

I will succeed on this plan because . . .

_____

_____

By now you're probably super excited to get to it, so let's jump in and blast off!

# PHASE 1—SHAKE IT UP (DAYS 1–3)

We've all managed to accumulate crud in our bodies that's blocking the absorption of nutrients from the food we eat, weighs us down with excess body fat, or deprives us of our energy. To remedy this, Phase 1 focuses on rebooting your body, so you can start with a clean slate and a clean engine; we'll "fire" like a well-oiled machine.

During the first three days, you enjoy a world of shakes, sweet and fruity as well as savory. Savory shakes are what I call soups! Each day of this phase, I give you four recipes: two sweet and two savory. You can enjoy these five to six times throughout your day. I'm not trying to torture or starve you, so make sure to drink as much as you need of these to feel satisfied. The shakes were carefully constructed to give you plenty of water, fiber, and a careful balance of fat-burning fats. Believe me when I say you'll get nice and full drinking these, so don't worry that you'll take in as many calories as you've been eating. Just focus on following the plan, and it will take you where you want to go.

Each of the recipes in Shake It Up includes several of our four Rocket Fuels, focusing on the ones with super anti-inflammatory, healthful enzymes, and detoxification benefits. Together they have the power to dissolve away the caked-on engine crud. I even give you the option to add on an additional "Squeaky Cleaner" ingredient that will help you Shake It Up even more to dislodge, let loose, and let go of accumulated toxins, junk, and body fat. Shake It Up and jettison the junk that's weighing you down.

During this phase, and all phases, you may also want to Shake It Up by getting your body moving. Again the diet is effective without exercise, but we both know that you can't be truly healthy if you sit on your bum all day. All you need is a brisk daily 20-minute walk to get your blood circulating and your heart pumping. Stretching is also beneficial; it will keep healthy oxygen flowing to all the cells in your body to help jettison deeply lodged fat and toxins out of your system. Saunas are a great thing to do during this phase, as well, if you have access to one.

# 15-Day Menu Plan

| DAY | Breakfast | Snack | Lunch |
|-----|-----------|-------|-------|
| 1 | Blueberry Blast | Pineapple Green Shake | Spicy Bok Choy Soup |
| 2 | Simple Strawberry Shake | Apple Green Mar-tea-ni | Ginger Soup |
| 3 | Pina Colada | Pear Power Shake | Spicy Avocado Soup |
| 4 | Ginger Mango Shake | Ginger Mango Shake (drink) or Grapefruit Salad (eat) | Easy Being Green Salad |
| 5 | Banana Shake | Banana Shake or Pomegranate Blueberry Salad | Spring Sauerkraut Salad with Thermo Dressing |
| 6 | Chocolate Banana Mylk Shake | Chocolate Banana Mylk Shake or Pineapple Coconut Salad | Asian Cabbage Salad with Apple Cider Vinaigrette |
| 7 | Matcha Shake | Matcha Shake or Pecan Candy Apple | Corn and Basil Mesclun Salad with Thermo Dressing or Apple Cider Vinaigrette |
| 8 | Vanilla Blueberry Shake | Vanilla Blueberry Shake or Red, White, and Blue Berry Salad | Kreamy Chipotle Salad with Kreamy Chipotle Dressing |
| 9 | Pineapple Cilantro Shake | Pineapple Cilantro Shake or Cucumber Guacamole | Cabbage Salad with Cucumber Miso Dressing |
| 10 | Pear Lime Ginger Shake | Pear Lime Ginger Shake or Watermelon Grapefruit Salad | Zucchini Hummus |
| 11 | Green Grapefruit Shake | Green Grapefruit Shake or Mint and Basil Tropical Fruit Salad | Shredded Sesame Salad with Orange Ginger Vinaigrette |
| 12 | Orange Vanilla Shake | Orange Vanilla Shake or Peach Crumble | Italian Salad |
| 13 | Avocado Shake | Avocado Shake or Fudge Brownie with Fresh Berries | Fennel Slaw with Dill Vinaigrette |
| 14 | Beauty Berry Shake | Beauty Berry Shake or Trail Mix Cookies | Cumin Slaw with Coconut Miso Vinaigrette |
| 15 | Choose shake | Choose shake or snack | Choose salad |

| Snack | Dinner | Snack |
|-------|--------|-------|
| Shake or soup | Tomato Bisque | Leftover soup |
| Shake or soup | Marvelous Minestrone | Leftover soup |
| Shake or soup | Curry Coconut Soup | Leftover soup |
| Strawberry Mint Shake | Red Pepper Soup | Soup, ½ avocado, or nuts |
| Pineapple Protein Shake | Kreamy Dill Delight | Soup, ½ avocado, or nuts |
| Mango Mint Shake | Coconut Tomato Soup | Soup, ½ avocado, or nuts |
| Smooth Operator | Souper Supper | Soup, ½ avocado, or nuts |
| Kreamy Cucumber Soup or Vanilla Blueberry Shake | Zucchini Noodles with Marinara Sauce | Soup, ½ avocado, or nuts |
| Garlic Bell Soup or Pineapple Cilantro Shake | Celery Almond Paté | Soup, ½ avocado, or nuts |
| Curried Cilantro Cucumber Soup or Pear Lime Ginger Shake | Mixed Vegetable Seaweed Rolls with Sesame Dipping Sauce | Soup, ½ avocado, or nuts |
| Coconut Miso Soup or Green Grapefruit Shake | Collard Rolls with Cashew Paté | Soup, ½ avocado, or nuts |
| Curried Zucchini Cucumber Soup or Orange Vanilla Shake | Marinated Mushrooms in Lettuce Wraps | Soup, ½ avocado, or nuts |
| Carrot Ginger Soup or Avocado Shake | Pesto Wraps | Soup, ½ avocado, or nuts |
| Kreamy Tomato Gazpacho or Beauty Berry Shake | Mushroom Rolls with Root Rice | Soup, ½ avocado, or nuts |
| Choose soup or shake | Choose soup or dinner meal | Soup, ½ avocado, or nuts |

## Double the Fun: Find a Partner

A great way to keep motivated is to have a weight-loss partner to keep you company during the next 15 days. You will provide each other with support. Being accountable to someone else makes a big difference in staying on track, and it's more fun to have another person with you committed to the same goals: getting lean, hot, and healthy!

## Simplified Recipe Option— For Those Who Really Feel Time-Stretched or Kitchen-Challenged

On this plan, I offer four shake recipes a day. But if you're traveling or you need to make up all your shakes in the morning to carry with you into a long workday, or if you just want to simplify things and do even less preparation on the plan, you can choose one of the sweet and one of the savory shakes and just triple up on the amounts you make. Then you can drink up and fill up on them throughout your day.

Enjoy sweet shakes during the first half of your day (breakfast and morning snack) and then switch to the savory soups for lunch, afternoon snack, and dinner.

During these three days, avoid chewing any solid foods. This may sound crazy at first, but don't worry, you'll still be eating. It's just that your blender will chew your food for you. The benefit of eating this way is that the nutrients are easier to absorb. You'll be taking in a ton of vitamins, minerals, enzymes, amino acids, and beneficial nutrients, while saving the energy usually spent chewing and breaking down your food. We're giving our digestive tract a break during this phase. This rest is naturally detoxifying because all that left-over energy instead cleanses and purges toxins lodged deep in our cells. We get a deep, squeaky clean, from the inside out.

## ⭐ Just Say No

Remember to enjoy beverages like water and green tea, but just say *no* to anything else, including coffee, alcohol, or diet soda for these 15 days.

# DAY 1 Shake It Up

Day 1 can be challenging, not because you'll be hungry because you won't. The idea of not eating can seem scary. Remember, though, you are eating. You're eating up a lot of nutrient-dense ingredients and letting the blender chew them all for you so you can rest, recover, and purge. This phase of the detox will get easier and easier each day. I promise. Besides, it's only three days. You can do this knowing that solid foods are just around the corner.

During any of the days of this plan, have more if you're still hungry! Raw Food is not about being hungry. Also, after dinner, if you find yourself hungry, feel free to have any leftover soup. But try not to eat after 7 p.m. or 8 p.m.

## Today's Menu

| | |
|---|---|
| BREAKFAST | **Blueberry Blast** |
| SNACK | **Pineapple Green Shake** |
| LUNCH | **Spicy Bok Choy Soup** |
| SNACK | *Shake or Soup* |
| DINNER | **Tomato Bisque** |
| SNACK | *Leftover soup (optional)* |

---

## ☆ POWER PACKED: *Cinnamon*

I think this sentence says it all; it's from Cinnamon and Health, a study published in October 2010, by Gruenwald et al, in a respected food science and nutrition journal: "Evidence suggests that cinnamon has anti-inflammatory, antimicrobial, antioxidant, antitumor, cardio-vascular, cholesterol-lowering, and immunomodulatory effects . . ."

That's a lot of punch for a little spice. Want to know just a pinch more? It also shows real promise in the treatment of type 2 diabetes.

*What challenged you today?*

_____

_____

_____

_____

*How do you feel?*

_____

_____

_____

_____

# DAY 2 Shake It Up

Congratulations, you've made it through Day 1 and into Day 2. I knew you could do it! You should notice, even with blending and preparing your shakes during the day, you have more time on your hands since you're not sitting down to eat a full meal. Use this extra time to take a brisk walk and/or stretch. Give your body some love!

As you progress through the plan, rate your recipes on a scale of 5 stars for your favorites to 1 star for your least favorites. Write the stars next to each recipe title. This will help you visually locate your favorite recipes with just a glance.

## 🖉 Clean Up Is a Whirl

A trick for cleaning your blender container is to fill it with water and a little soap, if using, and blend. Then rinse. That's it. Clean!

## Today's Menu

| | |
|---|---|
| BREAKFAST | **Simple Strawberry Shake** |
| SNACK | **Apple Green Mar-tea-ni** |
| LUNCH | **Ginger Soup** |
| SNACK | *Shake or Soup* |
| DINNER | **Marvelous Minestrone** |
| SNACK | *Leftover soup (optional)* |

*What challenged you today and how can you handle it differently/the same tomorrow?*

_____

_____

_____

_____

*What was easy?*

_____

_____

_____

_____

*How does your body feel?*

_____

_____

_____

_____

# DAY 3 Shake It Up

If you choose to make only two of the four shakes for the day, choose one sweet for the morning and one savory soup for the afternoon and evening. Make up triple batches. Store shakes in airtight, sealed containers for easy transport. Store in your fridge or in a cooler bag when traveling.

This is your final day on all shakes. Tomorrow, you'll start to include a green salad for lunch, and even a snack that you can bite into, if you find you need it. Hang in there! You're doing great, bravo!

## Today's Menu

| | |
|---|---|
| BREAKFAST | **Pina Colada** |
| SNACK | **Pear Power Shake** |
| LUNCH | **Spicy Avocado Soup** |
| SNACK | *Shake or Soup* |
| DINNER | **Curry Coconut Soup** |
| SNACK | *Leftover soup (optional)* |

*How was your day?*

_____

_____

_____

_____

*Have you noticed any physical changes since beginning this detox phase: weight loss, skin improvement, better digestion, better sleep?*

_____

_____

_____

_____

 **Staying in Orbit—Phase 1**

Here are some other tips to help you during the first three days of cleansing and detoxing because this can be the most challenging phase.

■ Get up and go for a walk around the block, your apartment, or even up and down your stairs whenever you find yourself craving food. You'll find out whether you're really hungry or just in need of a distraction.

■ Drink a glass of water with fresh-squeezed lemon (one or two wedges); it will help keep you hydrated. Plus, lemon is a super duper degreaser to help get your insides squeaky clean.

■ Since you're already cleaning out your body, why not occupy yourself with cleaning something else, like your fridge, car, closet?

■ Take a minute to meditate and keep any negative self-defeating thoughts and emotions in check. Take charge of your thoughts, direct them towards your goals, or even to God, Spirit, or the universal intelligence—whatever helps you keep the faith and focused on this path to health.

- Make sure to go to bed early enough so that you get a full night's sleep. The last thing you want during a cleanse or detox is to feel overtired or overworked.

- Take a long, hot bath or shower.

- Help someone in need by volunteering for a nonprofit, feeding the homeless, or helping out a neighbor. Helping others takes the focus off ourselves, helps us remember our blessings, and makes us feel good.

## PHASE 2—MELT DOWN (DAYS 4–7)

Congratulations! You've made it through Phase 1 and have successfully detoxed, rebooted, and are now squeaky clean. You should feel lighter, tighter, and you may find you've already lost several pounds. Most of my test group lost 3 to 5 lbs during Shake It Up! If all you have is 10 pounds to lose, you're already halfway there. I bet it has been easier than you thought it would be, yes?

Now, we're ready to move on to Phase 2, Melt Down, and jettison even more of those extra unwanted pounds and fat. During this phase, we introduce additional Rocket Fuels, with a laser focus on prebiotics and probiotics (the friendly 'Bots that will eat away belly fat) and MCFAs (the healthy fats we talked about earlier that dissolve and melt down unwanted body fat). In addition to the detoxing and cleansing ingredients from Phase 1, Phase 2 adds on additional beneficial 'Bot-containing fermented foods like sauerkraut, nutritional yeast, miso, apple cider vinegar, and capers. When you're at the health food store, pick up a few bottles of kombucha or kefir (water or coconut based). Avoid dairy during your 15 days. Drink a bottle a day to add even more beneficial belly-eating 'Bots! Brewing your own is simple; you can find recipes for Kombucha, Water Kefir, and Coconut Kefir in *Ani's Raw Food Essentials*, page 52 to 59.

During these next four days, you'll be adding back in solid foods during lunch and with your morning snack, if you choose. You'll continue to enjoy your shakes, smoothies, and soups for breakfast, afternoon snack, and dinner.

Use any spare time you have during this phase to be good to yourself, to chill out, while you give your body a chance to have a meltdown—a fat meltdown, that is!

## Repeat After Me

If you have more than 10 or 15 pounds to Melt Down, remember to repeat Phases 1 and 2 again for an additional week before moving on to Phase 3.

## Out to Lunch

Ideally, make your lunch and take it with you wherever you are heading. But if you're on the road, or don't have time to fix lunch, it's easy to find green salads at virtually any restaurant. Focus on whole vegetables and greens and avoid croutons, bread, heavy dressings, and sauces laden with empty calories.

When traveling and on the go, I love to carry sea vegetables, nuts, seeds, and nutritional yeast with me. (Trust me; the yeast tastes better than it sounds.) These ingredients all travel easily, take up little space, and make an easy add-on to any green salad to bump up flavor, nutritional profiles, and overall fat-melt-down power.

# DAY 4 Melt Down

If you're jetting along on shakes and smoothies and you feel you can continue with just shakes and a lunchtime green salad today, then go ahead. But, if you're feeling like you need to bite into something, enjoy a Grapefruit Salad for your morning snack, along with today's salad for lunch. Do whatever feels right for you. Take each day as it comes. Focus only on today, and worry about tomorrow, well, tomorrow. Or better yet don't worry about tomorrow. We all know stress can derail even our best intentions when it comes to eating and our health.

## Today's Menu

| | |
|---|---|
| BREAKFAST | **Ginger Mango Shake** |
| SNACK | **Ginger Mango Shake** |
| | *or* |
| | **Grapefruit Salad** |
| LUNCH | **Easy Being Green Salad** |
| SNACK | **Strawberry Mint Shake** |
| DINNER | **Red Pepper Soup** |
| SNACK | *Soup, ½ avocado, or a small handful of nuts (optional)* |

*Did you have any challenges today? What were they and how did you handle them?*

_____

_____

_____

_____

*How do you feel?*

_____

_____

_____

_____

# DAY 5 Melt Down

Check in with yourself to see how you feel today and give yourself what you need. Only you know what's right for you. Welcome with open arms (well, mouths) all those cute little belly-fat-eating 'Bots and thank them for helping melt down your body fat. Remember to mark your favorite recipes with 5 stars to make it easy to find them at a glance later.

## Today's Menu

| | |
|---|---|
| BREAKFAST | **Banana Shake** |
| SNACK | **Banana Shake** |
| | *or* |
| | **Pomegranate Blueberry Salad** |
| LUNCH | **Spring Sauerkraut Salad** *with* **Thermo Dressing** |
| SNACK | **Pineapple Protein Shake** |
| DINNER | **Kreamy Dill Delight** |
| SNACK | *Soup, ½ avocado, or a small handful of nuts (optional)* |

*What challenged you today, if anything?*

_____

_____

_____

_____

*After you finish this plan, what other new things will you try?*

_____

_____

_____

_____

# DAY 6 Take It Off

Consider making double and triple batches of the vinaigrette so you always have some on hand. You can even carry it with you in a small bottle if you want.

## Today's Menu

| | |
|---|---|
| BREAKFAST | **Chocolate Banana Mylk Shake** |
| SNACK | **Chocolate Banana Mylk Shake** <br> *or* <br> **Pineapple Coconut Salad** |
| LUNCH | **Asian Cabbage Salad** <br> *with* **Apple Cider Vinaigrette** |
| SNACK | **Mango Mint Shake** |
| DINNER | **Coconut Tomato Soup** |
| SNACK | *Soup, ½ avocado, or a small handful of nuts (optional)* |

*What challenged you today, if anything? What excited you today?*

_____

_____

_____

_____

*Write down five things that make you unique and special.*

_____

_____

_____

_____

_____

# DAY 7 Melt Down

You've just about reached the halfway mark. Congratulate yourself for taking care of yourself and challenging yourself to try something new! This is the final day of the Melt Down phase. People may be commenting by now that they notice you have an extra skip in your step. I bet you feel lighter, and I bet you've a little more room in your favorite skinny jeans, too. Notice how amazing you feel and strive to feel just as good, if not better, each and every day.

## Today's Menu

| | |
|---|---|
| BREAKFAST | **Matcha Shake** |
| SNACK | **Matcha Shake**<br>*or*<br>**Pecan Candy Apple** |
| LUNCH | **Corn and Basil Mesclun Salad**<br>*with* **Thermo Dressing or Apple Cider Vinaigrette** |
| SNACK | **Smooth Operator** |
| DINNER | **Souper Supper** |
| SNACK | *Soup, ½ avocado, or a small*<br>*handful of nuts (optional)* |

*List five things you did right today.*

_____

_____

_____

_____

_____

*Now that you've finished Phase 2, Melt Down, how much total weight have you lost? How do you feel? How does your skin look?*

_____

_____

_____

_____

### 🍃 Staying In Orbit—Phase 2

To keep you rocketing along your Blast Off plan, focus on small steps you're making each day to create a new habit that helps you to achieve your longer-term goal. Those small daily changes will add up over time to become a big change later.

- Replace negative habits with positive ones.

- Give yourself the days of your Phase 3, Blast Off, to undo an old habit while practicing a new one.

- Commit by telling everyone you know about your Blast Off and weight-loss goals. This will keep you accountable because you won't want to lose face.

- Reward yourself for a job well done each week. Perhaps you can take yourself to a movie, go for a massage, get a mani/pedi; do something that feels rewarding to you.

- Track your urges during and at the end of each day on this plan to become more aware of them. Write out a strategy so you have a plan for beating your urges next time they crop up. I find taking deep breaths and drinking water help me beat my urges.

- Track your progress during and at the end of each day so you can see your progress over these 15 days. It's motivating to see how far you've come. Consider posting your progress in a blog or sending e-mail messages to friends and family to keep you motivated and accountable.

- Think positive! When a negative thought creeps in, squash it immediately by replacing it with a positive thought instead. You can do this!! Think positive, and you will succeed.

- Accept "slip ups." If you fall off the raw foods wagon and find yourself in front of the fridge at 3 a.m., spoon in one hand and a pint of triple chocolate peanut butter ooze in the other, don't freak out. Don't use it as an excuse to give up. If you fall off, just jump right back onto the plan at your next snack or meal.

## PHASE 3—BLAST OFF (DAYS 8–15)

I'm so proud of you. You did it. You started this new mission and now are halfway through your journey. Step back for a moment and look at what you've accomplished in just a week.

During Phase 1, Shake It Up, you deep cleaned your engine using the Rocket Fuels that provide anti-inflammatory and cleansing power to get you rebooted to brand spanking shiny and new!

In Phase 2, Melt Down, you chose to fill your belly with powerful fat-eating 'Bots and fat-melting MCFA-packed fuels that melted down even more body fat.

Now, during your final Phase 3, Blast Off, you'll be rocket launching your success to the next level by adding on thermogenic (metabolism boosting) Rocket Fuels to blast off those final extra pounds. Remember these thermogenic foods were chosen specifically for their ability to raise body temperature, metabolism, and for their fat-burning benefits. Throughout this phase, you'll see that I highlight Thermo Chargers in the recipes that you can add to further boost your fat burning even more!

During this final phase, you'll continue to enjoy your unlimited shakes, soups, and salads as you did in Phase 2; plus now, you'll add on a delicious dinner meal, too.

During this final phase, you can increase your physical activity if you want. Perhaps a 20-minute jog, swim, or bike ride would feel good. For maximum fat burning results, I like to exercise longer than 35 minutes, even when walking, because the body starts to burn fat stores for energy after the first 35 minutes into a workout. Again, daily stretching is always a good habit.

# DAY 8 Blast Off

You get to have a lot of fun today. During this phase you get to stuff your face with the most delicious foods knowing that eating them will accelerate your weight loss. It's hard to imagine that chowing down can do this, but wait and see!

## Today's Menu

| | |
|---|---|
| BREAKFAST | **Vanilla-Blueberry Shake** |
| SNACK | **Vanilla-Blueberry Shake** |
| | *or* |
| | **Red, White, and Blue Berry Salad** |
| LUNCH | **Kreamy Chipotle Salad** |
| | *with* **Kreamy Chipotle Dressing** |
| SNACK | **Kreamy Cucumber Soup** |
| | *or* |
| | **Vanilla-Blueberry Shake** |
| DINNER | **Zucchini Noodles** *with* **Marinara Sauce** |
| SNACK | *Soup, ½ avocado, or small handful of nuts (optional)* |

*What challenged you today?*

_____

_____

_____

_____

*How do you feel?*

_____

_____

_____

_____

# DAY 9 Blast Off

To up thermogenesis with every sip, squeeze lemon into your water, maybe even add a pinch of cayenne, too. I like slicing cucumber and infusing that into my water. Drinking cold water will help you fill up, hydrate, and boost the detox process.

## Today's Menu

| | |
|---|---|
| BREAKFAST | **Pineapple Cilantro Shake** |
| SNACK | **Pineapple Cilantro Shake** |
| | *or* |
| | **Cucumber Guacamole** |
| LUNCH | **Cabbage Salad** *with* **Cucumber Miso Dressing** |
| SNACK | **Garlic Bell Soup** |
| | *or* |
| | **Pineapple Cilantro Shake** |
| DINNER | **Celery Almond Paté** |
| SNACK | *Soup, ½ avocado, or small handful of nuts (optional)* |

*What was your favorite part of your day? What can you do tomorrow to enjoy it even more?*

_____

_____

_____

_____

*Rate your energy levels. What fun thing can you do with that extra energy?*

_____

_____

_____

_____

## ⭐ POWER PACKED: *Sauerkraut and Pickles*

You can tell by now that I love fermented vegetables for their friendly fat-eating 'Bots . . . and for all the right reasons. And who knew the nation's favorite hot dog and hamburger toppings could pack such a great health punch? I did. And now you do, too. You may want to ditch the buns, the burgers, and the dogs, though. Cabbage is a powerful food on its own; sauerkraut, its fermented form, kicks it up a notch. What will eating these get you?

### Cabbage/Sauerkraut

- Protection against cancer (chemopreventive)
- Their probiotics are believed to enhance immune function, improve the function of the digestive tract, improve athletic performance (likely due to faster recovery from fatigue), and, of course, aid in weight loss.
- Lower cholesterol
- Great source of vitamins C and K

### Pickles/Cucumbers

- Great, glowing skin (substances in cukes—silica, ascorbic acid, and caffeic acid—all reduce irritation and swelling)
- Foods high in fiber, potassium, and magnesium can help to lower blood pressure.

# DAY 10 Blast Off

You're in the home stretch and almost two-thirds the way through your Raw Food Detox. Check back in with yourself by reading through your initial reasons for starting the plan and through your journal entries to date. You'll remember why you wanted to lose weight in the first place, which will increase your motivation if you find it flagging. Did you want to lose weight for an upcoming event, like a wedding, perhaps even your own wedding? Do you have a family or class reunion you're attending soon? Or did you just get sick of lugging around extra unwanted pounds? Whatever your motivation, applaud yourself for taking active steps to take care of you!

## Today's Menu

| | |
|---|---|
| BREAKFAST | **Pear Lime Ginger Shake** |
| SNACK | **Pear Lime Ginger Shake** |
| | *or* |
| | **Watermelon Grapefruit Salad** |
| LUNCH | **Zucchini Hummus** |
| SNACK | **Curried Cilantro Cucumber Soup** |
| | *or* |
| | **Pear Lime Ginger Shake** |
| DINNER | **Mixed Vegetable Seaweed Rolls** *with* **Sesame Dipping Sauce** |
| SNACK | *Soup, ½ avocado, or small handful of nuts (optional)* |

*What challenged you today, if anything?*

_____

_____

_____

_____

*How do you feel?*

_____

_____

_____

_____

# DAY **11** Blast Off

Don't forget to journal in the space I've created for you. Use that space each day; it's there for you. Use it today to begin a gratitude practice, if you'd like. Start by listing on paper 10 things you're thankful for. The first place I begin when doing this exercise is to give thanks for having all 10 toes. Staying in this space of gratitude helps me keep perspective and helps me avoid mindlessly trying to numb myself with food. Helping someone who is in need is a great way to kick-start your gratitude practice.

## Today's Menu

| | |
|---|---|
| BREAKFAST | **Green Grapefruit Shake** |
| SNACK | **Green Grapefruit Shake**<br>*or*<br>**Mint and Basil Tropical Fruit Salad** |
| LUNCH | **Shredded Sesame Salad**<br>*with* **Orange Ginger Vinaigrette** |
| SNACK | **Coconut Miso Soup**<br>*or*<br>**Green Grapefruit Shake** |
| DINNER | **Collard Rolls** *with* **Cashew Paté** |
| SNACK | *Soup, ½ avocado, or small*<br>*handful of nuts (optional)* |

*What are you grateful for today?*

_____

_____

_____

_____

*Who are you grateful for today?*

_____

_____

_____

_____

# DAY **12** Blast Off

Most people find it easier to exercise in the morning. I know I'm usually lacking the needed energy and motivation after a long workday to get myself up and at 'em. I just want to lie on my couch or rest by day's end. Working out first thing in the morning works best for me; it means I get my sweat on, my circulation pumping, and my metabolism revved up and burning on extra high all day long. Plus, I get it out of the way! And of course, if evening's your thing, if sunset really makes you want to head for a run or yoga, then use your twilight fitness to help you decompress before bed (I'm unable to work out late, as it wakes me up and keeps me from sleeping. But if it works for you, then great!). Regardless of the time of day, if you decide to do even a little something today, try a few push ups and lunges—no matter what the hour—to keep your body moving.

## Today's Menu

| | |
|---|---|
| BREAKFAST | **Orange Vanilla Shake** |
| SNACK | **Orange Vanilla Shake** |
| | *or* |
| | **Peach Crumble** |
| LUNCH | **Italian Salad** |
| SNACK | **Curried Zucchini Cucumber Soup** |
| | *or* |
| | **Orange Vanilla Shake** |
| DINNER | **Marinated Mushrooms in Lettuce Wraps** |
| SNACK | *Soup, ½ avocado, or small handful of nuts (optional)* |

*How was your day?*

_____

_____

_____

_____

*What do you want to be when you "grow up"? (Hey, this is your space to explore so why not dream big?)*

_____

_____

_____

_____

# DAY **13** Blast Off

Visualize your success; visualize your new self at your new ideal weight; you're almost there, so it shouldn't be too hard! Keep your mind focused on how great you feel now and how great you'll feel after you've blasted off all the baggage that's holding you down—both emotional and physical. Think about how great you will feel in your clothes or even what your new, smaller clothes will look like!

Remember, the main reason for weight loss is an expression of self-love; It's to benefit you, and only you. You're taking time and making the effort because you want to look and feel better. This is for you, and you deserve it!

## TODAY'S MENU

| | |
|---|---|
| BREAKFAST | **Avocado Shake** |
| SNACK | **Avocado Shake** |
| | *or* |
| | **Fudge Brownies** *with* **Fresh Berries** |
| LUNCH | **Fennel Slaw** *with* **Dill Vinaigrette** |
| SNACK | **Carrot Ginger Soup** |
| | *or* |
| | **Avocado Shake** |
| DINNER | **Pesto Wrap** |
| SNACK | *Soup, ½ avocado, or small handful of nuts (optional)* |

*What's the best you look like?*

_____

_____

_____

_____

*What's the best you feel like?*

_____

_____

_____

_____

# DAY **14** Blast Off

Do what you can to lessen the things that stress you. As we already know, stress increases production of that fat-promoting hormone, cortisol. When cortisol levels go up, we store belly fat, and that's not good. We can't avoid stress entirely in life, but how we frame and perceive our world affects whether we find it stressful or exciting. How will you look at your world? And when it's overwhelming what do you do to combat that feeling? The best remedy I've found to combat stress is exercise—even taking a break from work and stretching for 5 or 10 minutes can really help me feel energized and refocused. What works for you?

## Today's Menu

| | |
|---|---|
| BREAKFAST | **Beauty Berry Shake** |
| SNACK | **Beauty Berry Shake** |
| | *or* |
| | **Trail Mix Cookies** |
| LUNCH | **Cumin Slaw** *with* **Coconut Miso Sauce** |
| SNACK | **Kreamy Tomato Gazpacho** |
| | *or* |
| | **Beauty Berry Shake** |
| DINNER | **Mushrooms Rolls** *with* **Root Rice** |
| SNACK | *Soup, ½ avocado, or small handful of nuts (optional)* |

*Woohoo! One more day to go. How does that feel?*

_____

_____

_____

_____

*Now that you're almost through the 15 days, what changes have you noticed in your body? In your mind?*

_____

_____

_____

_____

# DAY 15

Celebrate! You've made it through the last two weeks of the 15-Day detox plan. Pat yourself on the back. Feel proud that you've allowed time for yourself and your health to be a priority.

To celebrate, you get to choose all of your favorite recipes to enjoy today. Beyond being a reward for all your dedication and hard work, this is designed to empower you to start thinking of ways you may like to incorporate the recipes you've learned here into the future and throughout the coming days, months, and years.

## Blast Off

Look over the recipe titles to find the ones you marked with 4 or 5 stars and choose your favorite recipes to enjoy today. Take time to notice how you feel right now. Read over your journal entries from the past two weeks and review your progress. Note all your challenges, along with all your positive changes.

Tomorrow, you'll be back to your normal routine and diet. This is your final day. Have a blast!

## Today's Menu

| | |
|---|---|
| BREAKFAST | *Choose any shake* |
| SNACK | *Choose any shake or snack* |
| LUNCH | *Choose any salad* |
| SNACK | *Choose any soup or shake* |
| DINNER | *Choose any soup or dinner meal* |
| SNACK | *Choose any favorite snack* |

*What will you eat tomorrow?*

_____

_____

_____

_____

*How will you continue to take care of yourself?*

_____

_____

_____

_____

*Is there anything you'd do differently next time?*

_____

_____

_____

_____

# 6

# THE RECIPES—Shakes, Salads, Soups, Rolls, Wraps, Noodles, and Desserts

Finally we have arrived at our launch pad and are ready to enjoy delectable recipes that will jettison weight loss. I've organized the recipes into the following sections so you can quickly thumb through and find what you need, when you need it.

Shakes

Salads

Soups

Rolls, Wraps, Noodles, and Patés

Desserts and Sweet Snacks

## GETTING AN ADDED BOOST

As you know, I've combined the Rocket Fuels together for maximum fat-blasting power and to support the specific goals of each of our three phases. But additional "power packs" may also be added to each meal to further charge it. The first three mentioned are phase-specific, but the last two can be used any time.

Squeaky Cleaner: foods or spices that add even more detoxifcation
and cell-cleansing power (Phase 1)

Fat Melter: foods with additional fat-eating 'Bots (Phase 2)

Thermo Charger: thermogenic foods that burn-baby-burn! (Phase 3)

Super Power Packed: Supercharged boosters are not required eating,
but they will max out your nutrient levels by adding in power-packed

foods like sea vegetables (including nori or wakame), blue-green algae like spirulina or chlorella, dehydrated grasses like barley grass powder or wheatgrass, and adaptogens like maca.

'Bot Boost: ingredients you should already have in your fridge that offer a way to add on even more belly-fat-eating 'Bots to a recipe.

Don't be afraid of these new foods and ingredients. All of them are easy to get and easy to use. If you don't have them at a local store, order them online at: www.GoSuperLife.com.

Also, you can replace the water in any of the shake recipes with the same amount of kefir or kombucha. Both are probiotic drinks packed with fat-eating 'Bots, and they are available at most natural food stores. These drinks can get expensive to buy, but they are really easy to make at home. I offer recipes for brewing your own cultured probiotic drinks like kefir and kombucha, even rejuvelac (a fermented, probiotic, grain drink) in *Ani's Raw Food Essentials*, pages 52 to 60.

## WHAT ELSE DO YOU NEED TO KNOW?

### SOME FINAL TIPS AND SUBSTITUTIONS

#### Bananas, pineapples, berries

I keep berries, peeled banana, and chunks of pineapple in the freezer to use in smoothies. This eliminates the need for ice and makes the smoothies cool and yummy.

#### Greens

Some shakes call for a particular green; some suggest a green but also say "or greens of your choice." If a recipe calls for kale, but you only have spinach, it is more than okay to use whatever you have on hand, or whatever you prefer taste-wise.

#### Soaking Your Nuts and Seeds

When using tree nuts and seeds, I recommend soaking them in filtered water overnight to allow them to begin germinating. In nature, a nut or seed is held dormant by an enzyme inhibitor, so a bird or animal will eat it and then expel it onto moist soil. Here, the nut or seed comes to life; it starts to germinate, preparing to grow a tree or plant. At this stage, the nut or seed contains higher levels of protein and lower levels of carbohydrates. And, as you read earlier in the book, they are also much easier to digest. Soaking nuts and seeds may seem cumbersome, but it's really simple! I like to soak whatever nuts and seeds I'll be using the following day in at least double the amount of water (1 cup nuts to 2 cups water, for example) before going to bed. The next morning, I rinse them well and discard the soaking water, which contains the enzyme inhibitors. I place the drained nuts and seeds in a bowl and shelve them uncovered in the fridge, where they begin to dry out. Ideally, I try to use these soaked nuts and seeds within a day or two. If I am unable to use them all, I'll dry them in a dehydrator set at 104 degrees for a few hours, until fully dry. If you don't have a dehydrator, you can set your oven on the lowest temperature and place soaked nuts and seeds on a baking tray until dry, maybe 20 minutes. Realize that using the oven means you're baking and cooking your soaked nuts and seeds. So, if you like the results, consider acquiring a food dehydrator; it dries at lower temperatures. Fully dried nuts and seeds will keep at room temperature for months and make for great travel food.

## WHAT IF YOU HAVE A TREE NUT ALLERGY?

I always choose whole foods first. But, for those who may have an allergy or intolerance to tree nuts, hemp protein powder or brown rice protein powder are great substitutes. You can get all of the substitutions listed below at www.GoSuperLife.com. Read on to learn how to use them.

### Hemp Protein

As you know from my earlier sidebar, hemp protein comes in a powdered form and is a great source of protein, fiber, and healthy fat. A 2-tablespoon serving has about 60 calories, 7 grams of carbohydrate, and 6 grams of protein. I like to mix hemp protein powder with equal parts flax meal to help mellow out the strong flavor of hemp. A 2-tablespoon serving of flax has about 70 calories, 2 grams of carbs, and 1 gram of protein; it is also a wonderful source of Omega 3s. To make flax meal, just grind flax seeds in a coffee grinder or high-speed blender.

The Switch: ¼ cup nuts for 2 tablespoons hemp protein powder + 2 tablespoons flax meal

## Sprouted Brown Rice Protein

You've heard about brown rice protein, but likely you haven't tried bio-fermented, sprouted brown rice protein, which is about 83 percent protein . . . wow! Two tablespoons has about 80 calories, 1 gram of fat, 5 grams of carbs, and 15 to 23 grams of protein depending on the manufacturer. Second to nuts, seeds, and sea vegetables, this is my favorite protein source.

The Switch: ¼ cup nuts for 2 tablespoons brown rice protein powder

# TAMING YOUR SWEET TOOTH

I've designed this plan to give you ample room to satisfy any sugar cravings you might have (as well as dessert salads throughout the plan to keep the sugar beast tamed). I know the best way to success is to stay with the plan, so I've done my best to make eating a treat here. Here's a little bit about the sweeteners used in the recipes, as well as other good choices for sweetening when you need a healthy sugar fix but still want to make the best choices for your health and waistline.

My favorite sweetener is stevia, a plant whose leaves have been dried into a green powder. Choose green stevia powder, when available, because it's less processed than the white powder or liquid form. Stevia is noncaloric and doesn't cause an insulin response in the body. Because it comes in a powder form, it works best added to liquids like shakes. Stevia has a strong flavor, and a pinch goes a long way.

Other sweeteners include syrups like honey, maple, palm, brown rice, and agave; each of these has about 60 calories per tablespoon. Honey is the least refined and is available in its raw form. Maple and palm syrup are minimally refined, made by extracting tree sap and boiling. I choose grade B maple syrup because it is less refined than grade A and contains more minerals and vitamins. Both honey and maple syrup are very sweet, so you don't need to use much in any recipe. Brown rice syrup is about half as sweet as table sugar, so you need to use more than other sweeteners, but it is popular for its complex sugars that are absorbed more slowly into the bloodstream. Agave has been touted as a healthy, low-glycemic sweetener, but today there is considerable debate about its high fructose content. Each of these syrups has varying consistencies and unique flavors, so personal preference and health goals will help you choose the one that's right for you.

From my unprocessed and whole food standpoint, the best sweeteners are always whole fruits. I make my own date syrup by blending pitted dates with water (recipe is on page 43 of *Ani's Raw Food Asia*). I include fruits like pineapple, bananas, dates, and berries to sweeten the recipes that follow.

If you prefer more sweetness, you can add one or two pitted dates. I prefer medjool dates for their flavor, semisoft texture, and large size. I'd rather that you use the sweetener of your choice, in moderation, if it will help you stick to our 15-day plan. The goal is for all my recipes to taste delicious and for you not to feel deprived.

The Sweet Switch: pinch of stevia = approximately 1 tablespoon syrup = 1 to 2 pitted dates

# SHAKES

## Apple Green Mar-tea-ni

**PHASE 1 SHAKE IT UP**
MAKES 1 PINT, 1 SERVING

This delicious morning shake is made by blending together apples with romaine lettuce and green tea to burn fat while increasing your metabolism. Add more cleansing power with ginger for an extra boost.

- 1 cup apple, seeded, diced, about 1 whole
- 1 cup romaine (or your favorite greens), torn, lightly packed, about 1 or 2 large leaves
- 1 cup brewed green tea (or ½ teaspoon matcha in 1 cup filtered water)

Additional water, as needed for desired consistency

**SQUEAKY CLEANER:**

1 teaspoon minced ginger, fresh

Place all ingredients, including ginger (if using), into your blender. Blend until smooth.

Will keep for two days in fridge.

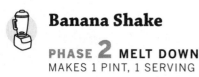

## Avocado Shake

**PHASE 3 BLAST OFF**
MAKES 1 PINT, 1 SERVING

Avocado is a fruit, rather than a vegetable, and it's commonly used in desserts and sweets in Southeast Asia. It adds heart-healthy fats, and a rich, creamy texture to recipes without adding cholesterol. The fat in the avocado and the fiber in the strawberries will fill you up in the morning and keep you satisfied longer. Drink up and kick off an awesome day!

1 cup strawberries, fresh or frozen

½ cup avocado flesh, from about ½ whole

pinch stevia powder, or 1 tablespoon of your favorite syrup, or 1 or 2 pitted dates, optional

1 cup filtered water

1 cup ice

**THERMO CHARGER:**

Replace filtered water with 1 cup brewed green tea,

*or*

½ teaspoon matcha powder in 1 cup filtered water.

**SUPER POWER PACK:**

Add ½ tablespoon of a super green like spirulina or wheatgrass powder.

Place all ingredients into your high-speed blender, including green tea and spirulina, if using. Blend until smooth.

Will keep two days in fridge.

## Banana Shake

**PHASE 2 MELT DOWN**
MAKES 1 PINT, 1 SERVING

I was inspired to create this recipe from a shake I tasted in Los Angeles that was made from bananas, a ton of almond butter, and cinnamon. It was so rich, really creamy, but too heavy. So I had to make my own version. Belly-blasting walnuts are high in good calories and healthy fat, plus researchers think the combination of protein, fiber, and healthy fats in nuts help keep you feeling full longer.

1 cup banana, from 1 medium whole

¼ cup walnuts (or 2 tablespoons hemp protein powder + 2 tablespoons flax meal, or 2 tablespoons brown rice protein powder)

¼ teaspoon ground cinnamon

1 cup filtered water

½ cup ice

**THERMO CHARGER:**

Substitute the water for 1 cup sun-brewed green tea, or ½ teaspoon matcha in 1 cup filtered water.

Place ingredients into a high-speed blender. Blend until smooth.

Best enjoyed immediately, but it will keep for one day in fridge.

## Beauty Berry Shake

PHASE **3** BLAST OFF
MAKES 1 PINT, 1 SERVING

Pumpkin seeds are a beauty secret I learned about from my Chinese medicine doctor. They're full of vitamin E, monounsaturated fatty acids (MUFAs), and are a great source of B vitamins and calcium, which provide beauty benefits for skin, hair, and nails. I love the way they taste, too.

1 cup strawberries or blueberries, fresh or frozen

¼ cup pumpkin seeds, raw, shelled

1 tablespoon virgin coconut oil

1 teaspoon vanilla extract, alcohol-free, or ½ whole vanilla bean

pinch stevia powder, or 1 tablespoon of your favorite syrup, or 1 to 2 pitted dates, optional

½ cup ice

½ to 1 cup filtered water, as desired

**THERMO CHARGER:**

**Replace filtered water with 1 cup brewed green tea**

*or*

**add ½ teaspoon matcha in 1 cup filtered water.**

Place all ingredients into your high-speed blender, including green tea, if using. Blend until smooth.

Will keep for two days in fridge.

## Blueberry Blast

**PHASE 1 SHAKE IT UP**
MAKES 1 PINT, 1 SERVING

It's simple to make a nut mylk by blending together water with your favorite nuts. I love fiber because it keeps me full and helps with cleansing. Some folks feel that almonds create a gritty texture when blended, which I don't mind. If it bothers you, though, you can always strain out the almond fiber using a filtration bag, or try using walnuts instead. Cinnamon is a thermogenic and an anti-inflammatory, and I love to enjoy this as my post workout shake.

**1 cup blueberries, fresh or frozen**

**¼ cup almonds or walnuts (or 2 tablespoons hemp protein powder + 2 tablespoons flax meal, or 2 tablespoons brown rice protein powder)**

**1 tablespoon virgin coconut oil**

**½ to 1 teaspoon ground cinnamon, to taste**

**½ cup ice**

**1 cup filtered water**

**THERMO CHARGER:**

**Substitute water in recipe for 1 cup brewed green tea,**

*or*

**½ teaspoon matcha powder in 1 cup filtered water.**

**SUPER POWER PACK:**

1 teaspoon spirulina

*or*

1 teaspoon chlorella powder

Place all ingredients, including green tea and spirulina, if using, into your high-speed blender. Blend until smooth.

Will keep for two days in the fridge.

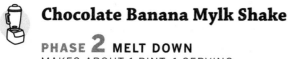

## Chocolate Banana Mylk Shake

PHASE **2** MELT DOWN
MAKES ABOUT 1 PINT, 1 SERVING

I was born in the year of the monkey, and I'm bananas for bananas. A ripe banana is a great sweetener. Add Omega 3-packed flax, chocolate, and green tea to pump up the fat-blasting power of this shake, and you're golden. Power-packed maca helps strengthen our adrenals to better handle stressors, while also making us stronger and healthier. I love enjoying this shake to fuel me up before a workout.

1 cup banana, about 1 whole

2 tablespoons flax seeds or meal

2 tablespoons cacao powder or cocoa powder

pinch stevia powder, or 1 tablespoon of your favorite syrup, or 1 to 2 pitted dates, optional

1 cup water, as desired

**THERMO CHARGER:**

Substitute the water with 1 cup green tea,

*or*

½ teaspoon matcha in 1 cup filtered water.

**SUPER POWER PACK:**

**1 to 2 teaspoons maca powder**

Place ingredients into a high-speed blender, including green tea and maca, if using. Blend until smooth.

Will keep for two days in fridge.

## Ginger Mango Shake

PHASE **2** MELT DOWN
MAKES 1 PINT, 1 SERVING

Mango, along with durian and leechee, is one of my favorite fruits. Almonds and mango blended together create a creamy base, while the coconut oil adds beneficial MCFAs for fat-blasting power and amazing flavor. If your mango is ripe, you won't need additional sweetener.

**1 cup mango, diced, fresh or frozen**

**¼ cup almonds (or 2 tablespoons hemp protein powder +
    2 tablespoons flax meal, or 2 tablespoons brown rice protein
    powder)**

**1 tablespoon virgin coconut oil**

**pinch stevia powder, or 1 tablespoon of your favorite syrup,
    or 1 to 2 pitted dates, optional**

**1 cup filtered water, for desired consistency**

**FAT MELTER:**

**1 teaspoon of fresh, grated ginger, to taste**

Place all ingredients, including ginger, if using, into your high-speed blender. Blend until smooth.

Will keep for two days in fridge.

# Green Grapefruit Shake

PHASE **3** BLAST OFF
MAKES 1 PINT, 1 SERVING

Grapefruit is a major Raw Food Detox ingredient. Paired with cucumber, cilantro, and lime, this shake becomes even more powerful and tasty. Omega 3s from flax, plus the MUFAs we love, make this shake one of my best fat-fighting friends, and now it's yours, too.

1 cup grapefruit, peeled and seeded, from about 1 small whole

½ cup cucumber, chopped, about ½ whole

2 tablespoons to ¼ cup cilantro or parsley, to taste

2 tablespoons lime juice, fresh, from about 1 whole

1 tablespoon flax meal

¼ teaspoon ground vanilla bean, or 1 tablespoon vanilla extract (alcohol-free), or ½ whole vanilla bean

½ cup ice

1 cup filtered water

**THERMO CHARGER:**

Replace 1 cup water with 1 cup green tea

*or*

add ½ teaspoon matcha powder.

**SUPER POWER PACK:**

1 to 2 tablespoons spirulina or wheatgrass powder

Place all ingredients into your high-speed blender, including green tea and spirulina, if using. Blend until smooth.

Will keep two days in fridge.

## Mango Mint Shake

PHASE **2** MELT DOWN
MAKES 1 PINT, 1 SERVING

Mango and mint is a favorite combo of mine. I experienced this pairing for the first time on a trip to Southeast Asia. This refreshing shake is packed with fiber, a vital ingredient for weight loss. Romaine lettuce is hidden inside this shake, a great way to up your vegetable intake.

**1 cup mango, diced, fresh or frozen**

**1 cup romaine, torn, about 1 to 2 large leaves**

**4 to 6 mint leaves, about 1 teaspoon, fresh, to taste**

**1 cup filtered water, as desired**

**FAT MELTER:**

**1 tablespoon virgin coconut oil**

Place ingredients into high-speed blender, including coconut oil, if using. Blend until smooth.

Will keep for one day in fridge.

## Matcha Shake

PHASE **2** MELT DOWN
MAKES 1 PINT, 1 SERVING

I love green tea and almond mylk in the morning. Blending together sun-brewed green tea, or powdered matcha with water, almonds, and banana makes this fat-blasting shake smooth and creamy.

**1 cup banana or 1 whole**

**¼ cup almonds (or 2 tablespoons hemp protein powder + 2 tablespoons flax meal, or 2 tablespoons brown rice protein powder)**

**1 cup brewed green tea, or ½ teaspoon matcha powder in 1 cup filtered water**

**½ cup ice**

**SUPER POWER PACK:**

1 teaspoon spirulina, or chlorella powder, and/or ½ teaspoon
   maca powder

Place all ingredients into your high-speed blender, including spirulina and maca, if using. Blend until smooth.

Will keep for two days in the fridge.

## Orange Vanilla Shake

PHASE **3** BLAST OFF
MAKES 1 PINT, 1 SERVING

This shake is inspired by the orange Creamsicles I remember loving as a kid. Packed with vitamin C and MCFAs, it's even more powerful if you add green tea. Plus, the spirulina or wheatgrass is a great source for protein and minerals.

1 cup orange, peeled and seeded and diced, from about 1½ whole

¼ cup almonds (or 2 tablespoons hemp protein powder +
   2 tablespoons flax meal, or 2 tablespoons brown rice protein
   powder)

¼ teaspoon ground vanilla bean, or 1 tablespoon vanilla extract,
   alcohol-free, or ½ whole vanilla bean

½ cup ice

½ to 1 cup filtered water, to desired consistency

**THERMO CHARGER:**

Add ½ teaspoon matcha powder or replace filtered water with
   1 cup brewed green tea.

**SUPER POWER PACK:**

½ to 1 tablespoon super green like spirulina or wheatgrass
   powder

Place all ingredients into a high-speed blender, including matcha and spirulina, if using. Blend until smooth.

Will keep two days in fridge.

## Pear Lime Ginger Shake

PHASE **3** BLAST OFF
MAKES 1 PINT, 1 SERVING

Pear adds fiber and whole-fruit sweetness, while lime and ginger increase the thermo power of this shake. Add pineapple for more sweetness and fat-melting action.

1 cup ripe pear, seeded and cubed, about 1 whole

juice of 1 lime (about 2 tablespoons)

1 tablespoon minced ginger

1 tablespoon virgin coconut oil

1 tablespoon flax meal

½ cup ice

1 cup filtered water

**FAT MELTER:**

¼ cup pineapple, diced, frozen or fresh

**THERMO CHARGER:**

Add ½ teaspoon matcha powder or substitute 1 cup brewed green tea instead of the water in the recipe.

Place all ingredients into your high-speed blender, including pineapple and green tea, if using. Blend until smooth.

Will keep two days in fridge.

## Pear Power Shake

PHASE **1** SHAKE IT UP
MAKES 1 PINT, 1 SERVING

I like blending together sweet fruits, like pear, with vanilla and kale to get more greens and fiber into my day for maximum detox benefit. Add on one or all of the Super Power Packs to up the shake's power; plus it adds more protein and more greens.

1 cup ripe pear, seeded and quartered, about 1 whole

1 cup kale, destemmed, torn

1 tablespoon vanilla extract, alcohol-free, or ½ whole vanilla bean

1 cup filtered water

½ cup ice

**SUPER POWER PACK:**

1 teaspoon spirulina, chlorella, or wheatgrass powder

Place all ingredients, including spirulina, if using, into your high-speed blender. Blend until smooth.

Will keep for two days in fridge.

 ## Piña Colada

PHASE **1** SHAKE IT UP
MAKES 1 PINT, 1 SERVING

Pineapple has a powerful proteolytic enzyme called bromelain that digests proteins, and it's used as a debriding agent to slough dead tissue from burns and wounds. It's also known to decrease inflammation, which is why it's a main ingredient during Days 1, 2, and 3.

1 cup pineapple, chopped, fresh or frozen

¼ cup almonds (or 2 tablespoons hemp protein powder +
    2 tablespoons flax meal, or 2 tablespoons brown rice protein
    powder)

1 tablespoon virgin coconut oil

1 tablespoon vanilla extract, alcohol-free, or ½ whole vanilla bean

1 cup filtered water

**SQUEAKY CLEANER:**

½ teaspoon matcha powder or 1 cup brewed green tea instead
    of 1 cup water

Place all ingredients into your high-speed blender, including green tea, if using. Blend until smooth.

Will keep for two days in fridge.

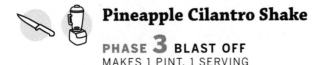

## Pineapple Cilantro Shake

**PHASE 3 BLAST OFF**
MAKES 1 PINT, 1 SERVING

Pineapple and cilantro sounded at first like a strange combo to me, but I gave it a try and was surprised at how much I liked the fresh flavors. Add cucumber, coconut, and flax for additional fat-blasting power.

- 1 cup pineapple, chopped, frozen or fresh
- ½ cup chopped cucumber, about ½ whole
- 2 tablespoons to ¼ cup fresh cilantro, chopped, to taste
- 1 tablespoon flax meal
- 1 tablespoon virgin coconut oil
- ½ cup ice
- 1 cup filtered water

**THERMO CHARGER:**

- Add ½ teaspoon matcha powder or replace filtered water above with 1 cup sun-brewed green tea.

Place all ingredients, including green tea, if using, into your high-speed blender. Blend until smooth.

Will keep two days in fridge.

## Pineapple Green Shake

**PHASE 1 SHAKE IT UP**
MAKES 1 PINT, 1 SERVING

When I first had sciatica in my right leg, I needed to decrease inflammation and pain quickly. So I made this shake with pineapple and flax, and it worked amazingly well.

- 1 cup pineapple, chopped, fresh or frozen
- 1 cup kale, loosely packed, about 1 leaf
- 1 teaspoon to 1 tablespoon fresh ginger, to taste
- 1 cup filtered water, or more, to desired consistency

**SQUEAKY CLEANER:**

Add a pinch of cayenne, to taste, or substitute 1 teaspoon turmeric for the ginger.

Place all ingredients into your high-speed blender, including cayenne, if using. Blend until smooth. Enjoy immediately.

Will keep two days in fridge.

## Pineapple Protein Shake

**PHASE 2 MELT DOWN**
MAKES 1 PINT, 1 SERVING

This shake saves me every time I have inflammation in my body from an injury or from a food sensitivity or intolerance. It removes puffiness and decreases swelling to make me leaner. It will help your body cool off during Melt Down, too!

1½ cups pineapple, chopped, fresh or frozen

1 tablespoon flax seeds or meal

1 cup filtered water, as desired

pinch stevia powder, or 1 tablespoon of your favorite syrup, or 1 to 2 pitted dates, optional

**SUPER POWER PACK:**

1 teaspoon spirulina or chlorella

Place ingredients, including spirulina, if using, into high-speed blender. Blend until smooth.

Will keep for two days in fridge.

## Simple Strawberry Shake

**PHASE 1 SHAKE IT UP**
MAKES 1 PINT, 1 SERVING

I love waking up on a summer morning and whipping up this simple shake. It's packed with antioxidants and low-glycemic strawberries for a beautiful red color. Cashews and coconut round out the flavor profile, and the vanilla just makes it pop. When strawberries are fresh and in season, you won't need to add additional sweetener. Frozen berries give a great consistency, but they aren't as sweet, so add a touch of your favorite sweetener if you'd like.

1 cup strawberries, fresh or frozen

¼ cup cashews or walnuts, ideally soaked in filtered water overnight and rinsed well

1 tablespoon virgin coconut oil

1 tablespoon vanilla extract, alcohol-free, or ½ whole vanilla bean

pinch stevia powder, or 1 tablespoon of your favorite sweetener like agave, maple or brown rice syrup, optional

½ cup ice

1 cup filtered water

**SQUEAKY CLEANER:**

Add ½ teaspoon matcha to the 1 cup filtered water in the recipe or replace the water with 1 cup brewed green tea instead.

Place all ingredients into your high-speed blender, including green tea, if using. Blend until smooth.

Will keep for two days in fridge.

## Strawberry Mint Shake

**PHASE 2 MELT DOWN**
MAKES 1 PINT, 1 SERVING

I love using avocado in my shakes because it gives them creamy richness. Add in strawberries and mint to mask the kale to help you get in more greens. Delicious!

1 cup strawberries, fresh or frozen

½ cup kale, any type, or your favorite greens

¼ cup avocado, about ¼ whole

2 tablespoons fresh mint

pinch stevia powder, or 1 tablespoon of your favorite syrup, or 1 to 2 pitted dates, optional

1 cup filtered water, as needed for desired consistency

**FAT MELTER:**

⅛ to ¼ teaspoon cayenne, or pinch to taste

Place ingredients into high-speed blender, with cayenne, if using. Blend until smooth.

Best enjoyed immediately, but it will keep for one day in fridge.

## Smooth Operator

**PHASE 2 MELT DOWN**
MAKES 1 SERVING

Move over sodium-laden, factory-produced vegetable drinks and canned soups. Resin linings in tin cans contain Bisphenol-A, aka BPA, linked to reproductive problems, heart disease, diabetes, and obesity. A study by the Harvard School of Public Health, reported in the *New York Times* on December 11, 2011 by Tara Parker-Pope in her column on Health, demonstrated that eating canned soup for one week increased BPA levels in subjects by over 1,200 percent! Instead try this flavor-packed and nutrient-rich alternative.

1 cup chopped tomatoes

½ cup chopped celery

½ cup chopped romaine

1 teaspoon ginger, grated

2 teaspoons miso, unpasteurized, any color

1½ cups filtered water

**FAT MELTER:**

½ to 1 teaspoon fresh garlic, minced

Place all ingredients into your high-speed blender, including garlic, if using. Blend until smooth.

Will keep two days in fridge.

# Vanilla Blueberry Shake

**PHASE 3 BLAST OFF**
MAKES 1 PINT, 1 SERVING

Blueberries taste amazing with vanilla. I like to use ground vanilla pods for fresh aroma and flavor. Green tea and ice are your thermogenics here. Add in some wheatgrass or spirulina, and you'll be blasting off, big time.

- **1 cup blueberries, fresh or frozen**
- **¼ cup almonds or walnuts (or 2 tablespoons hemp protein powder + 2 tablespoons flax meal, or 2 tablespoons brown rice protein powder)**
- **1 cup brewed green tea**
- **¼ teaspoon ground vanilla bean, 1 tablespoon vanilla extract, alcohol-free, or ½ whole vanilla bean**
- **½ cup ice**
- **1 cup filtered water**

**SUPER POWER PACK:**

**Drink 1 oz wheatgrass juice before having the shake**

*or*

**add 1 to 2 tablespoons of spirulina or wheatgrass powder to the shake before blending.**

Place all ingredients, including spirulina, if using, into your high-speed blender. Blend until smooth.

Will keep two days in fridge.

# SALADS

 **Asian Cabbage Salad
with Apple Cider Vinaigrette**

**PHASE 2 MELT DOWN**
MAKES 1 SERVING

This salad is full of prebiotics that will help the 'Bots eat up your belly fat.
I created this salad to be reminiscent of Southeast Asia by using the simple,
fresh, bright flavors of fresh mint, cilantro, and basil. It's colorful and pretty.

Add on nutritional yeast for a cheesy flavor sprinkle. One ounce of nutritional
yeast contains 14 grams of protein and 79 calories and is a great alternative
to animal proteins.

   2 cups shredded Napa cabbage, or green cabbage, loosely packed

   1 cup shredded carrot, about 1 whole

   ¼ cup cucumber, sliced thinly into half-moons

   1 tablespoon mint leaves, freshly torn

   1 tablespoon fresh cilantro leaves

   2 teaspoons basil leaves, freshly torn

   2 tablespoons almonds, whole

   **'BOT BOOST:**

   1 tablespoon nutritional yeast

## APPLE CIDER VINAIGRETTE

MAKES 2 SERVINGS

A quick and easy basic vinaigrette I like to use when I'm in a hurry or just feeling lazy. It's packed with probiotics from the vinegar. I recommend making a couple batches and keeping it in a jar in the fridge, just like we keep bottled, store bought dressings. Ready to eat—only better!

**2 teaspoons apple cider vinegar**

**3 tablespoons extra virgin olive oil, or 2 tablespoons olive oil and 1 tablespoon flax or hemp oil**

**½ teaspoon sea salt**

**Pinch black pepper**

To make the salad, place all salad ingredients in a mixing bowl.

To make the vinaigrette, whisk together ingredients in small bowl.

To serve, toss salad with **Apple Cider Vinaigrette**. Finish it with a sprinkling of nutritional yeast, if using, to add a cheesy flavor.

⭐ **What the Heck is Nutritional Yeast?**

A deliciously cheesy-flavored flaky powder that is found at most health food stores, often times in the bulk food section, nutritional yeast is a great protein source containing about 52 percent protein. It has essential amino acids, is gluten free, is rich in B-complex vitamins, and is a great source of folic acid. Nutritional yeast is specifically grown for its nutritional value. It's grown on a mix of cane and beet molasses for seven days, and B-vitamins are added during the process to give the yeast the nutrients it needs to grow. It's low in fat and salt, is kosher, non-GMO, and contains no added sugars or preservatives. One heaping tablespoon contains 60 calories, 1 gram of fat, and 8 grams of protein. Nutritional yeast should not be confused with active dry yeast or brewer's yeast.

I love sprinkling heaping tablespoons of nutritional yeast over my soups and salads, in my wraps, and on my noodles and kale chips to add a parmesan-cheese flavor and texture.

# Cabbage Salad
# with Cucumber Miso Dressing

**PHASE 3 BLAST OFF**
MAKES 1 SERVING

Think a salad can only be made with lettuce greens? Then think again and chomp on this. Cucumber Miso Dressing was inspired by one of my popular packaged food dressings, created for SmartMonkey Foods®. You'll love this recipe.

**2 cups cabbage, shredded**

**½ cup carrots, shredded**

## CUCUMBER MISO DRESSING

MAKES 1 CUP

**1 cup cucumber, diced, about 1 small**

**2 tablespoons miso, unpasteurized, any color**

**1 tablespoon ginger, minced**

**1 tablespoon toasted sesame oil**

**1 tablespoon extra virgin olive oil**

**2 tablespoons apple cider vinegar**

**THERMO CHARGER:**

**1 tablespoon nutritional yeast**

**SUPER POWER PACK:**

**1 tablespoon dulse flakes**

To make the salad, place cabbage and carrots into a mixing bowl.

To make the dressing, whisk together all dressing ingredients in a small bowl.

To serve, pour as much dressing as desired onto cabbage and toss until all is well-coated. Top with nutritional yeast and dulse flakes, if using.

Tossed salad will keep for a couples days. Dressing will keep up to one week in a sealed container, ideally glass, in the fridge.

# Corn and Basil Mesclun Salad

PHASE **2** MELT DOWN
MAKES 1 SERVING

Spring greens, radishes, sweet corn kernels, and fresh basil. Beautifully colored and prebiotic-rich, these make up a delicious and delicate salad. Toss it with either the Thermo Dressing or Apple Cider Vinaigrette, or another dressing you have on hand from this plan.

**2 cups spring green mix, or your favorite mesclun greens**

**3 radishes, sliced**

**¼ cup corn kernels, fresh**

**1 tablespoon basil leaves, torn**

**FAT MELTER:**

**½ to 1 teaspoon fresh ginger, minced**

Place all ingredients into a mixing bowl, including ginger, if using.

To serve, toss with either **Thermo Dressing** or **Apple Cider Vinaigrette**, pages 138 or 130.

Tossed salad is best enjoyed immediately.

# Cumin Slaw with Miso Vinaigrette

PHASE **3** BLAST OFF
MAKES 3 CUPS, 1 SERVING

Cabbage is abundant in vitamins C and E, calcium, magnesium, potassium, and iodine and is known for its many health benefits including helping with weight loss, and skin, eye, hair, and brain health. I enjoy eating and juicing both purple and green cabbage daily.

**2 cups cabbage, shredded, any type**

**½ cup cucumber, diced**

**½ cup tomato, diced**

½ cup carrot, shredded

1 tablespoon scallions, sliced

1 tablespoon cumin seeds

Place slaw ingredients into a bowl.

To serve, toss with **Coconut Miso Vinaigrette**.

## COCONUT MISO VINAIGRETTE

MAKES ABOUT ¼ CUP

Miso is one of my favorite fermented foods. It's high in protein, rich in flavor, and adds a great saltiness to recipes. This dressing is packed with probiotics from the apple cider vinegar, too, as well as MCFAs from the coconut oil for amazing mouth feel and flavor.

2 tablespoons virgin coconut oil

2 tablespoons miso, unpasteurized, any color

1 tablespoon apple cider vinegar

To make dressing, mix ingredients together in a small bowl using a fork or spoon.

Dressing will keep for many weeks in your fridge. The coconut oil will harden in the fridge, so warm the dressing to room temperature before using by placing in a bowl of hot water, or take it out and place on your counter an hour before using.

## Easy Being Green Salad

PHASE **2** MELT DOWN
MAKES 1 SERVING

This is the quickest and easiest dressing-free salad recipe ever! Greens are tossed with avocado for creaminess and sauerkraut and capers for probiotic tart-salty goodness. Corn and tomatoes add a touch of sweetness and beautiful colors.

2 cups spinach, lightly packed

1 cup red leaf lettuce, torn, about 2 to 3 leaves

½ cup avocado, about ½ whole

½ cup sauerkraut, drained

1 teaspoon capers, drained

2 tablespoons corn kernels, fresh

2 tablespoons chopped tomatoes or handful of grape or cherry
   tomatoes

**FAT MELTER:**

⅛ to ¼ teaspoon cayenne pepper, or a pinch, to taste

Place spinach and lettuce in mixing bowl. Add avocado, and mix well using
your hands to massage avocado into the greens and coat them evenly. You
can always just dice the avocado and toss with salad tongs if you prefer.
Me, I love to touch my food. Next, add sauerkraut and capers and mix well.
Top with corn and tomato.

Best enjoyed immediately, but it will keep for one day in fridge.

# Fennel Slaw with Dill Vinaigrette

**PHASE 3 BLAST OFF**
MAKES 3 CUPS, 1 SERVING

Filled with some of my favorite Rocket Fuels, this dish is a great starter, side,
or snack when you're craving something crunchy, salty, and sweet.

2 cups fennel, shredded

1 cup jicama, shredded

2 tablespoons sunflower or pumpkin seeds

**THERMO CHARGER:**

pinch black pepper, to taste

**'BOT BOOST:**

1 tablespoon nutritional yeast

## DILL VINAIGRETTE

MAKES ABOUT ¼ CUP

1 tablespoon apple cider vinegar

1 tablespoon virgin coconut oil

1 tablespoon fresh dill, chopped

1 teaspoon miso, unpasteurized, any color

¼ teaspoon lemon zest

To make the slaw, place fennel, jicama, and seeds in large mixing bowl.

To make the dressing, whisk together vinegar, coconut oil, dill, miso, and zest.

To serve, toss slaw with dressing, black pepper, and nutritional yeast, if using, and mix well.

Tossed slaw will keep up to three days in fridge. Vinaigrette will keep for a week or longer stored in air tight container, ideally glass, in fridge.

## Italian Salad

PHASE **3** BLAST OFF
MAKES 3 CUPS, 1 SERVING

A nongreen salad made instead with tomatoes, avocado, olives, basil, oregano, and scallions. Coconut oil gives you some great MCFAs, and apple cider vinegar provides the fat-eating 'Bots we love.

2 cups tomatoes, diced, from about 2 whole

1 cup avocado, cubed, from about 1 whole

3 tablespoons black olives, seeded, chopped

3 tablespoons fresh basil leaves, julienned

1 tablespoon scallions, sliced

1 tablespoon virgin coconut oil

2 teaspoons fresh oregano leaves

2 teaspoons apple cider vinegar

**THERMO CHARGER:**

⅛ teaspoon black pepper, or a pinch, to taste

**'BOT BOOST:**

1 tablespoon nutritional yeast

*and/or*

1 tablespoon capers

Place all ingredients, including black pepper, nutritional yeast, and capers, if using, into a mixing bowl. Toss to mix well.

Best enjoyed immediately, but it will keep up to one day in fridge.

## Kreamy Chipotle Salad

PHASE **3** BLAST OFF
MAKES 1 SERVING

This recipe is inspired by a vegan junk food version of a chipotle mayo that I just love. It's so simple to make a healthy, whole food recipe, instead. And this is hands down one of my favorite dressings.

**3 cups romaine and red leaf lettuce, shredded**

**¼ cup cucumber, sliced**

**3 tablespoons red bell pepper, diced**

**2 tablespoons celery, diced**

### KREAMY CHIPOTLE DRESSING

MAKES 1 CUP

**1 cup cashews, soaked in filtered water for 6 to 8 hours, rinsed well, and drained**

**1 tablespoon miso, unpasteurized, any color**

**¼ teaspoon chipotle, to taste**

**½ to ¾ cup filtered water, to desired consistency**

**THERMO CHARGER:**

**1 tablespoon nutritional yeast**

To make salad, place salad ingredients together in a mixing bowl.

To make dressing, place dressing ingredients into a high-speed blender. Blend until smooth.

To serve, pour as much dressing as desired over greens and toss gently. Best served immediately.

Dressing will keep stored separately for one week or longer in fridge.

# Shredded Sesame Salad
# with Orange Ginger Vinaigrette

**PHASE 3 BLAST OFF**
MAKES 1 SERVING

Who says that sesame makes a great flavor addition to most any salad? Says me! Sesame seeds have essential fatty acids and are high in mono-unsaturated fats to stimulate and boost metabolism.

1 ½ cups cabbage, shredded, any type

½ cup carrot, shredded, about ½ whole

¼ cup cucumber, julienned, about ¼ whole

3 tablespoons red bell pepper, julienned, about ⅙ whole

2 tablespoons celery, julienned, about ¼ whole

## ORANGE GINGER VINAIGRETTE

**PHASE 3 BLAST OFF**
MAKES 1 CUP

1 teaspoon fresh ginger, grated

1 to 2 teaspoons nama shoyu or braggs or tamari, to taste

2 teaspoons apple cider vinegar

¼ cup fresh orange juice, squeezed from about 1 whole

**THERMO CHARGER:**

1 teaspoon sesame seeds

**SUPER POWER PACK:**

¼ cup dry seaweed, like wakame or arame, soaked and drained

To make salad, place all salad ingredients into a large mixing bowl.

To make dressing, whisk ingredients together in a small bowl to blend well.

To serve, toss salad with as much dressing as desired. Top with sesame seeds and seaweed, if using. Enjoy.

Tossed salad will keep for a couple days in fridge. Dressing will keep four or five days in fridge when stored separately in a sealed container, ideally glass.

# Spring Sauerkraut Salad with Thermo Dressing

PHASE **2** MELT DOWN
MAKES 1 SERVING

Before you get scared off the idea of using sauerkraut in a salad, give this recipe a try. The varied textures and tastes make it both a nutritional power-house and a tasty dish. Promise.

3 cups spring mesclun mix, or your favorite greens

½ cup sprouts, any type

⅓ cup sauerkraut

2 tablespoons seeds or nuts (sunflower seeds, almonds, walnuts, whole)

## THERMO DRESSING

MAKES 1 CUP, 6 TO 8 SERVINGS

½ cup extra virgin olive oil, or ¼ cup virgin olive oil and ¼ cup hemp or flax oil

¼ cup apple cider vinegar

¼ cup miso, unpasteurized, any color

1 to 2 teaspoons ginger, minced, fresh, to taste

1 tablespoon nama shoyu (raw soy sauce)

**FAT MELTER:**

pinch black pepper, to taste

**'BOT BOOSTER:**

1 tablespoon nutritional yeast

To make the salad, place all salad ingredients into a large mixing bowl.

To make dressing, place its ingredients into high-speed blender or smaller personal blender. Blend until smooth.

To serve, toss salad with dressing. Sprinkle on black pepper and nutritional yeast, if using, and enjoy. Tossed salad is best enjoyed immediately. Dressing will keep for a couple weeks, or longer, when stored separately in fridge.

# SOUPS

## Carrot Ginger Soup

**PHASE 3 BLAST OFF**
MAKES 2 CUPS, 1 SERVING

I love cooked carrot ginger soup, and I created this raw recipe when I had a craving for it. Easy-to-blend carrots are joined by probiotic miso, thermogenic ginger, and creamy avocado for a dose of beneficial MUFAs.

1 cup carrot, chopped, about 1 whole

½ cup avocado, from about ½ whole

1 tablespoon miso, unpasteurized, any color

1 teaspoon ginger, minced

1 cup filtered water, as desired

**THERMO CHARGER:**

1 teaspoon virgin coconut oil

*or*

⅛ teaspoon chipotle powder, to taste

Place all ingredients, including coconut oil and chipotle, if using, into high-speed blender. Blend until smooth. Enjoy immediately.

Soup will keep in fridge for two to three days stored in sealed container, ideally glass.

## Coconut Miso Soup

**PHASE 3 BLAST OFF**
MAKES 2 CUPS, 1 SERVING

A light miso broth made with MCFA-rich coconut oil and thermogenic ginger, this soup is great as a light snack or paired with any meal.

> 2 tablespoons miso, unpastuerized, any color
>
> 1 tablespoon virgin coconut oil
>
> 1 teaspoon ginger, grated
>
> 2 cups filtered water

**THERMO CHARGER:**

> ⅛ teaspoon cayenne powder or a pinch, to taste

**SUPER POWER PACK:**

> 1 tablespoon dry wakame, rehydrated in water for five minutes, then squeezed to remove excess water

Whisk together miso, oil, ginger, water, and cayenne, if using, or place these ingredients into high-speed blender and blend smooth.

To serve, scoop into a soup bowl. Top with hydrated wakame, if using. Enjoy.

Will keep in an airtight container in the fridge for three to four days, or longer.

## Coconut Tomato Soup

**PHASE 2 MELT DOWN**
MAKES 1 PINT, 1 SERVING

I had this soup on my first visit to Phuket, Thailand. I'd never thought to pair the flavors of tomato and coconut, but I was wowed by the combination. This recipe makes for a delicious twist on regular tomato soup or gazpacho. Because I like garlic I'll add ¼ teaspoon of it to this soup. Feel free to add less, to suit your taste.

> 2 cups tomatoes, chopped from about 2 whole
>
> 1 tablespoon virgin coconut oil

1 tablespoon miso, unpasteurized, any color

½ to 1 teaspoon fresh ginger, grated

**FAT MELTER:**

⅛ to ¼ teaspoon garlic, minced, to taste

Place ingredients, including garlic, if using, into high-speed blender. Blend until smooth.

Will keep for three days in fridge.

## Curried Cilantro Cucumber Soup

PHASE **3** BLAST OFF
MAKES 1 PINT

I love making raw soups because they're so quick to whip together, and you can enjoy them like a savory shake or spoon them up in a bowl. Curry powder gives this soup an Asian flare.

1 cup cucumber, peeled, diced, about 1 whole

½ cup tomato, diced, about ½ whole

½ cup avocado, about ½ whole

2 tablespoons cilantro, fresh

1 tablespoon virgin coconut oil

1 teaspoon curry powder

1 teaspoon miso, unpasteurized, any color

1 cup filtered water

**THERMO CHARGER:**

⅛ teaspoon cayenne powder, or a pinch, to taste

Place all ingredients, including cayenne, if using, into high-speed blender. Blend until smooth. Enjoy immediately.

Will keep in fridge for three to four days, or longer, when stored in airtight container.

## Curry Coconut Soup

PHASE **1** SHAKE IT UP
MAKES 1 PINT, 1 SERVING

I like the flavor of coconut. Added to a splash of tart lemon, Asian curry, cilantro, avocado, and tomato . . . wow!

1 cup avocado, diced, about 1 whole

1 cup tomato, diced, about 1 whole

1 tablespoon lemon juice, from about ¼ whole

1 tablespoon virgin coconut oil

1 tablespoon fresh cilantro

¼ to ½ teaspoon curry powder

1 teaspoon miso, unpasteurized, any color

1 cup filtered water

**SQUEAKY CLEANER:**

¼ teaspoon minced fresh garlic

Place all ingredients, including garlic, if using, into your high-speed blender. Blend until smooth.

Will keep in fridge for one day when stored in airtight container, ideally glass.

## Garlic Bell Soup

PHASE **3** BLAST OFF
MAKES 1 PINT, 1 SERVING

Make this soup for a party and you'll be the "bell" of the ball. It's that good.

2 cups red bell pepper, diced, about 1 whole large

½ cup avocado, from about ½ whole

2 tablespoons lemon juice, fresh, from about ½ whole

1 tablespoon miso, unpasteurized, any color

½ teaspoon garlic, crushed, about 1 clove

½ to 1 cup filtered water, as desired

**THERMO CHARGER:**

1 teaspoon virgin coconut oil

*and/or*

⅛ teaspoon chipotle powder, to taste

Place all ingredients, including coconut oil and chipotle, if using, into a high-speed blender. Blend until smooth. Best enjoyed immediately.

Will keep, well-covered, in fridge for one or two days.

## Ginger Soup

PHASE **1** SHAKE IT UP
MAKES 1 PINT, 1 SERVING

Great for fighting a cold but also just plain yummy, this soup can be served cold or warm, if preferred. As with all of our soups, you can leave it blending a bit longer to heat slightly. Its lemon is great for flushing out toxins and unwanted bacteria from your body.

1 cup spinach, loosely packed

1 cup cucumber, chopped

½ cup avocado, about ½ medium whole

1 tablespoon lemon juice, from about ¼ whole

1 tablespoon miso, unpasteurized, any color

1 teaspoon to 1 tablespoon ginger, to taste

1 to 2 cups of filtered water, as desired

**SQUEAKY CLEANER:**

¼ to ½ teaspoon curry or turmeric powder

Place all ingredients, including curry, if using, into a high-speed blender. Blend until smooth.

Will keep for one or two days in fridge stored in airtight container, ideally glass.

## Spicy Bok Choy Soup

**PHASE 1 SHAKE IT UP**
MAKES 1 PINT, 1 SERVING

Avocado is one of my favorite foods. Not only does it taste great, but because of its healthy fat content, eating it helps you absorb more nutrients from certain foods, particularly the carotenoids. It is also a great source of glutathione, the "master" antioxidant, and it's the best fruit source for vitamin E.

**1 cup bok choy, chopped, loosely packed (or your favorite greens)**

**1 cup cucumber, diced, from about 1 whole**

**½ cup avocado, from ½ whole**

**1 tablespoon lemon juice, about ¼ whole**

**1 tablespoon miso, unpasteurized, any color**

**¼ jalapeño pepper, or pinch cayenne powder, to taste**

**1 to 2 cups of filtered water, for desired consistency**

**SQUEAKY CLEANER:**

**1 tablespoon ginger**

*or*

**1 tablespoon turmeric**

*or*

**pinch black pepper, to taste**

Place all ingredients, including ginger or turmeric or black pepper, if using, into your high-speed blender. Blend until smooth.

Best enjoyed immediately, but soup will keep for one day in an airtight container in the fridge.

## Kreamy Tomato Gazpacho

**PHASE 3 BLAST OFF**
MAKES 2 CUPS, 1 SERVING

You might not think that blending almonds in a tomato soup would work too well, but think again. These health-promoting beauties, combined with the coconut oil, give this gazpacho a creamy richness that is to live for!

1 cup tomato, chopped, about 1 whole, any type

¼ cup almonds, chopped

1 tablespoon virgin coconut oil

1 tablespoon miso, unpasteurized, any color

¼ to ½ teaspoon garlic, minced, to taste

1 cup filtered water, as desired

**THERMO CHARGER:**

⅛ teaspoon cayenne powder, to taste,

*or*

¼ fresh jalapeño pepper, to taste

Place all ingredients, including cayenne or jalapeño, if using, into a high-speed blender. Blend until smooth. Enjoy immediately.

Soup will keep in fridge for at least three to four days sealed in airtight container.

## Curried Zucchini Cucumber Soup

PHASE **3** BLAST OFF
MAKES 2 CUPS, 1 SERVING

I like to think of blended soups as savory shakes. I love this soup because the zucchini blended with the miso gives it a creamy base, while the lemon adds a touch of acidity and brightness.

½ cup zucchini, chopped, about 1 small whole

½ cup cucumber, chopped, about ½ whole

½ cup celery, chopped, about 1 rib

1 tablespoon lemon juice, from about ¼ whole

1 tablespoon miso, unpasteurized, any color

¼ teaspoon curry powder, to taste

1 cup filtered water, as desired

pinch cayenne powder, to taste,

*and/or*

½ teaspoon garlic, about 1 clove

Place all ingredients, including cayenne and garlic, if using, into your high-speed blender. Blend until smooth. Enjoy immediately.

Will keep for one day in fridge stored in sealed container.

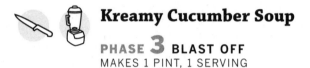

## Kreamy Cucumber Soup

**PHASE 3 BLAST OFF**
MAKES 1 PINT, 1 SERVING

When I spell the word *cream*, I like to use a *k* because it denotes a vegan version, without the dairy cream. It's oh so dreamy, too. Holy cow!

1½ cups romaine lettuce, torn, loosely packed, about 2 large leaves, or your favorite greens

1 cup cucumber, chopped, from about 1 whole

1 teaspoon fresh lemon juice, about ¼ whole

1 tablespoon miso, unpasteurized, any color

½ cup avocado, from about ½ whole

1 cup filtered water, as desired

**FAT MELTER:**

1 teaspoon virgin coconut oil

**THERMO CHARGER:**

⅛ teaspoon chipotle powder, to taste

Place all ingredients, including coconut oil and chipotle, if using, into a high-speed blender. Blend until smooth. Enjoy immediately.

While best enjoyed immediately, this soup will keep, well-sealed, in the fridge for one day.

## Kreamy Dill Delight

PHASE **2** MELT DOWN
MAKES 1 PINT, 1 SERVING

Blending together cashews with water makes a smooth, rich, kream. To this kream base we blend green spinach and broccoli, probiotic miso for saltiness, and dill for flavor.

**1 cup spinach, chopped, loosely packed**

**½ cup broccoli, chopped**

**¼ cup cashews, chopped**

**2 teaspoons miso, unpasteurized, any color**

**1 teaspoon dill, dry, to taste, or 2 teaspoons fresh, to taste**

**1 cup filtered water, for desired consistency**

**FAT MELTER:**

**1 tablespoon lime juice, about ½ whole**

Place ingredients, including lime juice, if using, into a high-speed blender. Blend until smooth.

Will keep for two days in the fridge stored in sealed container, ideally glass.


## Marvelous Minestrone

PHASE **1** SHAKE IT UP
MAKES 1 PINT, 1 SERVING

I've always loved minestrone soup and the flavors of Italian spices. Instead of salt, I use miso for its probiotic belly-fat eating 'Bots, as well as the more traditional garlic and oregano for bold flavor in this blended soup.

**1 cup tomato, diced, about 1 whole**

**1 cup celery, diced, about 2 ribs**

**1 tablespoon miso, unpasteurized, any color**

**½ teaspoon fresh oregano, or ¼ teaspoon dry**

**¼ teaspoon fresh garlic, minced**

⅛ to ¼ teaspoon cayenne, to taste

½ to 1 cup filtered water, as desired

**SQUEAKY CLEANER:**

½ tablespoon hemp or flax oil

Place all ingredients in a high-speed blender, including hemp oil, if using. Blend until smooth. Enjoy.

Recipe will keep for three or four days in the fridge when stored in a tightly sealed container, ideally glass.

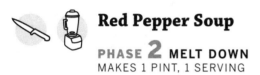

# Red Pepper Soup

PHASE **2** MELT DOWN
MAKES 1 PINT, 1 SERVING

Sprouts are like baby power plants that are high in protein and oxygen, and they are alkalinizing, rather than acidifying to our body, which is something we want. I like to add sprouts to my wraps, salads, and soups for texture, flavor, and of course, nutrients.

1 cup red bell pepper, diced, about 1 whole

½ cup sprouts, any type, loosely packed

½ cup avocado, about ½ whole

1 tablespoon lemon juice, from about ¼ whole

1 tablespoon miso, unpasteurized, any color

1 teaspoon basil, fresh or ½ teaspoon dry

1 cup filtered water, as desired

**FAT MELTER:**

¼ teaspoon chipotle powder, to taste

**SUPER POWER PACK:**

1 teaspoon dulse seaweed, whole or flakes

Place ingredients, including chipotle and dulse, if using, into a high-speed blender. Blend until smooth.

Best enjoyed immediately, but soup will keep for one day, well-covered, in the fridge.

# Souper Supper

PHASE **2** MELT DOWN
MAKES 1 PINT, 1 SERVING

When I make soups, I love to add fiber to them with cucumber and celery because both vegetables have mild flavors. Avocado adds a smooth kreaminess, and miso adds a savory saltiness. To mix it up, I like to use whatever fresh or dry herbs I may be craving that day, or I'll use dill because I like it with cucumber.

1 cup cucumber, diced, about 1 whole

1½ cup celery, chopped, about 2 whole ribs

½ cup avocado, about ½ whole

½ tablespoon fresh lemon juice, from about ¼ whole

2 tablespoons miso, unpasteurized, any color

2 teaspoons fresh dill, or your favorite herb, or 1 teaspoon dry

1 to 2 cups filtered water, as desired

**FAT MELTER:**

½ jalapeño pepper, or more, to taste

*or*

¼ teaspoon cayenne powder, to taste

*or*

pinch black pepper, to taste

Place all ingredients, including pepper, if using, into your high-speed blender. Blend until smooth.

Best enjoyed immediately, but soup will keep in an airtight container for one day in the fridge.

## Spicy Avocado Soup

PHASE **1** SHAKE IT UP
MAKES 1 PINT, 1 SERVING

This recipe was inspired by a craving I had for a rosemary version of guacamole while I was following a detoxifying cleanse. The avocado is filling and satisfying, and the smoky chipotle adds a great flavor profile.

**1 cup avocado, from about 1 whole**

**1 tablespoon miso, unpasteurized, any color**

**1 tablespoon fresh lime juice, from about ½ whole**

**¼ teaspoon fresh rosemary or ⅛ teaspoon dry**

**1 pinch chipotle powder, to taste**

**1 to 2 cups filtered water, to desired consistency**

**SQUEAKY CLEANER:**

**1 teaspoon virgin coconut oil**

Place all ingredients into your high-speed blender. Blend until smooth.

Best enjoyed immediately, but soup will keep in fridge for a half to a full day stored in an airtight container.

## Tomato Bisque

PHASE **1** SHAKE IT UP
MAKES 1 PINT, 1 SERVING

Not only yummy, this soup has at its center, the tomato. Recent research suggests that tomatoes, besides being a good source of fiber and lycopene, also help regulate the hormone ghrelin, one of the hormonal messengers responsible for telling us that we're full.

**1 ½ cups tomatoes, chopped**

**½ cup avocado, about ½ whole**

**½ teaspoon garlic, chopped**

½ teaspoon fresh thyme or ¼ teaspoon dry

½ teaspoon sea salt

1 cup filtered water, for desired consistency

**'BOT BOOST:**

**Serve sprinkled with 1 teaspoon to 1 tablespoon of nutritional yeast.**

Place all ingredients into your high-speed blender. Blend until smooth. To serve, sprinkle with nutritional yeast, if using. Enjoy.

Will keep for one day in fridge.

# ROLLS, WRAPS, NOODLES, PATÉS

 **Collard Rolls with Cashew Paté**

PHASE **3** BLAST OFF
MAKES 2 ROLLS

Collards offer a great way to wrap up your favorite fillings to make a hand-held delight. In this recipe, the collard is used like a flour tortilla would be, and it's filled with a delicious, nutritious, cashew paté. These rolls travel well, too.

1 large collard green leaf

1 avocado, peeled, seeded, sliced

1 cucumber, sliced into long strips

2 scallions, sliced into long strips, optional

1 batch **Cashew Paté**, below

## CASHEW PATÉ

MAKES ABOUT 1 CUP

½ cup cashew meal (process whole, dry cashews into a powder; set aside)

½ cup celery, chopped

1 teaspoon apple cider vinegar

½ teaspoon garlic, minced, about 1 small clove

1 tablespoon miso, unpasteurized, any color

**SUPER POWER PACK:**

1 teaspoon dulse flakes

To make paté, place celery, vinegar, garlic, miso, and dulse, if using, into food processor. Process into small pieces. Add cashew meal and process to mix well.

To make rolls, first remove stem from collard leaf. You will have two halves. Use each half leaf to make one roll, for a total of two rolls.

Place each half leaf flat. Top with ¼ cup paté across shorter width of leaf, a few slices of avocado, cucumber, and scallions, if using. Roll up leaf lengthwise. Enjoy immediately.

Leftover paté will keep for a day or two in the fridge.

## Marinated Mushrooms in Lettuce Wraps

PHASE **3** BLAST OFF
MAKES 1 SERVING

This recipe is inspired by a popular Korean BBQ meat dish but is made using mushrooms instead. It is super simple to make and amazingly delicious to eat! Mushrooms have been used in Chinese medicine for thousands of years to help restore our body's balance and natural resistance to disease. They're a great protein source, too.

### MUSHROOMS

1 tablespoon tamari or nama shoyu or soy sauce

½ tablespoon agave, maple, or brown rice syrup

1 teaspoon toasted sesame oil

1 cup sliced shiitake, crimini, or portabella mushrooms

**SUPER POWER PACK:**

1 teaspoon dulse flakes

### WRAPS

**4 lettuce leaves, like iceberg or red lettuce**

**1 tablespoon white miso, unpasteurized**

**½ cup (total) carrot and cucumber, julienned**

**½ jalapeño pepper, thinly sliced**

Marinate your **Mushrooms** by placing tamari, agave, and sesame oil into a large mixing bowl. Add mushrooms and dulse flakes, if using, and toss to mix well. Set aside to marinate 10 minutes or longer. Squeeze out excess liquid before serving.

Next, make **Wraps** by laying each lettuce leaf flat. Spread about ¼ tablespoon miso across center of each leaf. Top with marinated mushrooms, carrot, cucumber, and pepper, as desired. Enjoy immediately.

Will keep for a day in the fridge. Marinated mushrooms will keep for up to five days in fridge when stored separately.

## Mixed Vegetable Seaweed Rolls with Sesame Dipping Sauce

**PHASE 3 BLAST OFF**
MAKES 2 ROLLS, 1 SERVING

Sushi anyone? This is my delicious vegan spin on the traditional roll.

**2 nori sheets, untoasted, raw**

**2 tablespoons miso, unpasteurized, any color**

**2 cups sprouts, any type**

**½ cup avocado, sliced, about ½ whole**

**¼ cup cucumber, julienned, about ¼ whole**

**¼ cup carrot, julienned, about ½ whole**

Spread 2 teaspoons of miso, to taste, across the edge of 1 nori sheet. Layer sprouts, avocado, cucumber, and carrot across the same edge, up to about ⅓ the nori sheet. Roll up nori to enclose fillings. Lay on seam to keep roll closed.

Serve immediately with **Sesame Dipping Sauce**.

Will keep for one day in fridge stored in a sealed container. The nori will be soggy.

## SESAME DIPPING SAUCE

1 tablespoon nama shoyu, tamari, or soy sauce

1 tablespoon apple cider vinegar

1 teaspoon toasted sesame oil

1 teaspoon scallions, sliced

**THERMO CHARGER:**

¼ teaspoon cayenne, to taste

To make sauce, whisk together all ingredients, including cayenne, if using. Mix well.

Sauce will keep for a week or longer stored in an airtight container in fridge.

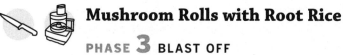

# Mushroom Rolls with Root Rice

**PHASE 3 BLAST OFF**
MAKES 1 SERVING

Marinating mushrooms in tamari will help them wilt and "cook" down after about 10 minutes. This concentrates the flavor as it would if you were to sauté them while cooking.

## MUSHROOMS

1 tablespoon tamari, or nama shoyu, or soy sauce

½ tablespoon agave, maple, or brown rice syrup

1 teaspoon toasted sesame oil

1 cup mushrooms, sliced, any type

**SUPER POWER PACK:**

1 teaspoon dulse flakes

Marinate **Mushrooms** by placing all ingredients, including dulse, if using, into a mixing bowl, toss and massage to mix well. Set aside to marinate at least 10 minutes. Squeeze to remove all excess liquid before using.

## ROOT RICE

MAKES ABOUT 1 CUP

This looks just like traditional rice, has a similar mouth feel, and is great to use just as you would regular cooked rice.

**1 cup jicama, turnip, or daikon radish, peeled and cubed**

**½ tablespoon white miso, unpasteurized**

**2 teaspoons scallions, sliced, from about 1 whole**

Chop jicama, miso, and scallions into small pieces in food processor. Be careful not to over process; you want small rice-sized bits.

Rice will keep for several days in sealed container in fridge.

## WRAPS

The collard leaf in these wraps helps to create a moisture barrier that keeps the nori on the outside dry.

**2 sheets nori paper**

**1 collard leaf, destemmed, and cut into 2 halves, towel-dried**

**½ cup (total) carrot and cucumber, julienned**

To make **Wraps**, lay down nori paper and place ½ collard leaf along edge closest to you (to create moisture barrier between fillings and nori paper). Top collard with about ¼ cup rice, about ¼ cup mushrooms, carrots, and cucumber. Roll upward and away from you. Cut into six pieces using a very sharp knife. Enjoy immediately.

Will keep for one day in fridge, but nori paper will get soggy. Best to store ingredients separately and assemble them before eating. Mushrooms and rice will keep for at least four days in fridge.

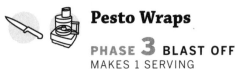 ## Pesto Wraps

PHASE **3** BLAST OFF

MAKES 1 SERVING

Pesto is simple to make, and most traditional pestos are already raw, minus the cheese that goes into some recipes. You can add nutritional yeast to add a cheesy flavor here. I use lower-fat pistachios rather than pine nuts, but the garlic and basil give it that familiar pesto flavor. Rather than oil in this recipe, I use avocado instead for its healthy fat-blasting fat.

## PESTO

½ cup pistachios, shelled and raw

1 teaspoon garlic, minced, about 1 medium-sized clove

1 tablespoon miso, unpasteurized, any color, to taste

1 cup basil, fresh, lightly packed

2 teaspoons lemon juice, about ½ whole

¼ cup avocado

### THERMO CHARGER:

Add 1 to 2 tablespoons nutritional yeast, to taste.

### SUPER POWER PACK:

Add 1 teaspoon dulse flakes.

## WRAPS

1 large collard leaf, destemmed and cut into 2 halves

¼ cup cucumber, diced

¼ cup red bell pepper, diced

¼ cup sprouts, any type

To make **Pesto**, chop pistachios into small pieces in food processor. Add remaining ingredients, including nutritional yeast and dulse, if using, into food processor, and process to mix well. Set aside.

Next, make **Wraps** by laying both half leaves flat. Spread about ¼ cup pesto across shorter direction. Top with cucumber, pepper, and sprouts. Roll up and enjoy immediately.

Wraps will keep for a day in fridge. Pesto will keep for four to five days stored separately in a sealed container in fridge.

## Celery Almond Paté

PHASE **3** BLAST OFF
MAKES 2 CUPS

Scoop this onto a bed of greens, wrap it in a sheet of nori or in a collard leaf, or scoop it up with sticks of celery. You can also shape the paté into patties and dehydrate them if you choose. They make a great snack or appetizer, while providing a good 'Bot boost.

1½ cups celery, chopped, about 3 ribs

½ tablespoon fresh ginger, grated

½ teaspoon fresh garlic, minced, about 1 clove

¼ cup raisins

1 tablespoon miso, pasteurized, any color

½ cup almond meal (process dry almonds into a powder and set aside)

1 teaspoon fresh herbs (dill, tarragon, oregano)

Place celery, ginger, garlic, raisins, and miso into a food processor. Process into small pieces. Be careful not to over process; you want small bits but not a slurry. Add almond meal and pulse to mix. Add in fresh herbs of your choice, if using, and pulse lightly to mix.

Serve with carrot and celery sticks, or rolled into a nori or collard wrap.

Pate will keep for three or four days stored in an airtight container in fridge.

## Cucumber Guacamole

PHASE **3** BLAST OFF
MAKES 2 CUPS, 1 SERVING

My friend Alex, who was once a contestant on Bravo's *Top Chef*, came over one day to make guacamole with me. This is what we came up with as an alternative to traditional guacamole, and it's super yummy.

1 cup avocado, about 1 whole, cut roughly

½ cup cucumber, thinly sliced, about ½ whole

½ tablespoon lemon juice, from about ⅛ whole

¼ teaspoon garlic, about 1 small clove

⅛ teaspoon sea salt, to taste

**THERMO CHARGER:**

pinch cayenne pepper, to taste

Place all ingredients, including cayenne, if using, into a bowl and mix well, leaving chunks of avocado. You want a chunky texture, rather than smooth.

Best enjoyed immediately.

To store, press firmly into a storage container. Cover with plastic wrap, removing all air pockets. Seal with the container lid.

Will keep for one day in the fridge.

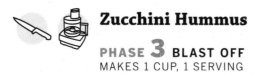 ## Zucchini Hummus

**PHASE 3 BLAST OFF**
MAKES 1 CUP, 1 SERVING

Enjoy this dish as a dip for carrots, celery sticks, and asparagus spears on a bed of greens, or wrapped in a leaf or sheet of nori.

¼ cup cashews

½ teaspoon garlic, minced, about 1 clove

1 cup zucchini, from about 1 whole

1 tablespoon fresh lemon juice, from about ¼ whole

1 tablespoon miso, unpasteurized, any color

**'BOT BOOST:**

2 tablespoons nutritional yeast

First, place cashews and garlic into a food processor. Process into small pieces. Next, add zucchini, lemon juice, miso, and nutritional yeast, if using, and process to mix well. You know it's ready when you have a creamy hummus consistency.

Will keep for four to five days in fridge stored in an airtight container.

# Zucchini Noodles with Marinara Sauce

**PHASE 3 BLAST OFF**
MAKES 1 SERVING

If you're craving a pasta dish, try this healthy variation instead. This makes a great centerpiece for a meal or a terrific side dish.

## NOODLES:

1 zucchini, cut into 4-inch chunks, about 1 cup
*or*
1 bag of kelp noodles, rinsed and drained well

To make noodles, use a spiralizer to cut zucchini into angel hair noodle strips. If you don't have a spiralizer, you can cut long strips shaped like fettuccini noodles instead. Place noodles into a large mixing bowl. Or, if using the kelp noodles, pop them into a mixing bowl and rinse very well first, and then drain well before using. Set aside.

## MARINARA SAUCE

MAKES 1 PINT, 4 SERVINGS

This fresh marinara can be tossed with vegetable or kelp noodles and also used as a dressing on a green salad. The lycopene in the tomatoes is great for your brain, and the olive oil is good for your heart. So eat up!

1½ cups cherry tomatoes

2 teaspoons fresh oregano, or 1 teaspoon dried

½ teaspoon fresh rosemary, or ¼ teaspoon dry

1 tablespoon lemon juice, from ¼ whole

¼ cup extra virgin olive oil

½ teaspoon sea salt, to taste

### THERMO CHARGER:

½ teaspoon garlic, about 1 small clove

To make **Marinara Sauce**, place all ingredients, including garlic, if using, into your high-speed blender. Blend until smooth.

To serve, spoon sauce over **Zucchini Noodles** or kelp noodles, and top with basil and rosemary.

# DESSERTS AND SWEET SNACKS

 **Fudge Brownies with Fresh Berries**

PHASE **3** BLAST OFF
MAKES 4 SERVINGS

I love raw desserts because they are guilt-free and healthy! Imagine, you can have your cake and eat it, too. Really, no joke. This recipe makes four servings for most, which is more like one or two servings for me! I recommend doubling up on this recipe so you always have these on hand to snack on when you're in need of a dessert fix.

1 cup dry walnuts

¼ cup cacao powder or carob powder

pinch sea salt, to taste

⅓ cup medjool dates, pitted

½ cup fresh raspberries or strawberries

**SUPER POWER PACK:**

¼ teaspoon maca powder, to taste

To make **Brownies**, combine walnuts, cacao powder, salt, and maca, if using, in food processor. Pulse into medium pieces. Use some of this mix to powder the bottom of a baking pan. Add dates and pulse to mix well. Batter should stick together when squeezed into a ball. If it's too loose, add a few more sticky dates to help bind it together or a splash of filtered water. If it's too sticky, add a few more crushed dry walnuts to firm it up.

Scoop brownie mix into the powdered baking pan and flatten it to about ½ inch to ¾ inch thick by pressing lightly. Cut it into squares.

To serve, place brownie on serving dish and top with berries.

Brownies will keep for a few weeks or longer in the fridge when stored in a sealed container separate from the berries.

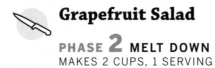

## Grapefruit Salad

PHASE **2** MELT DOWN
MAKES 2 CUPS, 1 SERVING

A lovely refreshing treat and great source of vitamin C, this salad is simple, delicious, and nutritious—the perfect dessert or snack.

**2 cups grapefruit wedges, seeded, from about 1 whole**

**1 teaspoon ground cinnamon**

**FAT MELTER:**

**½ to 1 teaspoon fresh ginger, slivered, to taste**

Place grapefruit pieces in a bowl, sprinkle with cinnamon and ginger. Enjoy immediately.

Will keep for a day in the fridge (but you won't want to wait to eat this one).

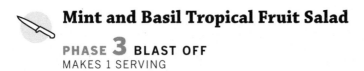

## Mint and Basil Tropical Fruit Salad

PHASE **3** BLAST OFF
MAKES 1 SERVING

Grapefruit is low in calories and high in enzymes that burn fat. Served with strawberries and banana, it makes for a confetti of color. Add fresh herbs for a full-speed celebration for your taste buds.

1 cup grapefruit, diced, from about 1 small whole

½ cup strawberries, sliced

½ cup banana, sliced, about ½ whole

1 teaspoon fresh mint, julienned

1 teaspoon fresh basil, julienned

¼ teaspoon fresh ginger, grated

**SUPER POWER PACK:**

Add ¼ to ½ teaspoon maca powder, to taste,

*and/or*

¼ teaspoon bee pollen, optional (only if you're not allergic to bees or sensitive to pollen).

Place all ingredients into a serving bowl and gently toss. To serve, top with maca and bee pollen, if using.

Salad will keep for one to two days in fridge stored in an airtight container.

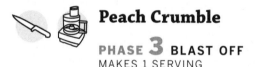

## Peach Crumble

PHASE **3** BLAST OFF

MAKES 1 SERVING

A simple crumble crust is made with pecans and dates, plus coconut oil for a buttery mouth feel and flavor. Use this crumble to top your favorite sliced fruit, and voila, it's become a beautiful dessert! It's super easy and fast. Plus, the crumble keeps well out of the fridge and makes for great travel food.

If it's not peach season, substitute your favorite fruit like apples, berries, or persimmons.

### CRUST

⅓ cup pecans

⅛ teaspoon sea salt

¼ cup medjool dates, pitted

1 teaspoon virgin coconut oil

### FILLING

2 cups peaches, sliced, from about 2 whole

¼ teaspoon vanilla powder, or 1 tablespoon vanilla extract, alcohol-free

**SUPER POWER PACK:**

¼ teaspoon maca powder, to taste

To make crust, combine pecans and salt in food processor. Pulse into medium-sized pieces. Add dates and coconut oil, and pulse to mix well. Texture should be sticky but also crumbly at the same time. If the mixture is too loose, add a splash of water or more dates; if it's too sticky, add more pecans.

To make filling, toss peach slices with vanilla.

Assemble in serving bowl by sprinkling half of the crust into bottom of bowl. Next, add peaches. Then, top with crust. Gently pat down, and enjoy.

Peach Crumble will keep for a few days in fridge. Store crumble crust separately, and it will keep for weeks in the fridge in an airtight container.

## Pecan Candy Apple

**PHASE 2 MELT DOWN**
MAKES 1 SERVING

A simple way to spruce up slices of apples with crushed pecans, vanilla, and a hint of cinnamon for a delicious dessert or sweet snack. Yum.

1 ½ cups apple, seeded, cored, diced

2 tablespoons pecans, crushed

1 teaspoon ground cinnamon

1 tablespoon vanilla extract, alcohol-free, or ½ whole vanilla bean

**FAT MELTER:**

1 teaspoon virgin coconut oil

**THERMO CHARGER:**

pinch black pepper, to taste

Place apples and pecans in a mixing bowl. Toss with cinnamon and vanilla and coconut oil, if using. Sprinkle on a pinch of black pepper, if using. Serve.

Will keep for one day in fridge before apples begin oxidizing. Store in airtight container.

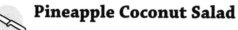

## Pineapple Coconut Salad

PHASE **2** MELT DOWN
MAKES 1 SERVING

Who said salad can't be a dessert? Like a trip to the tropics, this simple recipe explodes with flavor and bursts with health-promoting goodness.

**2 cups fresh pineapple, diced, about ½ whole**

**2 tablespoons dried coconut, shredded**

**FAT MELTER:**

**1 to 2 teaspoons fresh ginger, grated**

Place pineapple in bowl, and sprinkle coconut and ginger on top, if using.

Will keep for two to three days in fridge. Store in airtight container.

## Pomegranate Blueberry Salad

PHASE **2** MELT DOWN
MAKES 1 SERVING

Forget about wasting money on premade pomegranate juice. You'll get all the benefit for a whole lot less money by eating this sweet salad. If you can't find pomegranate, substitute either blackberries or strawberries.

**1½ cup blueberries**

**½ cup pomegranate seeds**

**2 teaspoons flax meal**

**¼ teaspoon ground cinnamon**

**FAT MELTER:**

**1 tablespoon cacao nibs**

Place blueberries and pomegranate into a serving bowl. Top with flax meal, cinnamon, and cacao nibs, if using.

Will keep for two days in fridge.

## Red, White, and Blue Berry Salad

**PHASE 3 BLAST OFF**
MAKES 1 SERVING

My amazing marathon-running athlete friend made this recipe for me, and I just loved it. Packed with low-glycemic, antioxidant-rich berries, and topped with crunchy cacao nibs for energy and flax for Omega 3s, it doesn't get much easier or yummier than this!

1½ cup fresh strawberries, sliced

½ cup fresh blueberries

1 tablespoon cacao nibs

2 teaspoons flax meal

**THERMO CHARGER:**

¼ to ½ teaspoon maca powder, to taste,

*and/or*

1 teaspoon bee pollen (if allergic to bees or honey,
     please do not add)

Place berries into a serving bowl. Top with cacao nibs, flax meal, and, if using, the maca and bee pollen.

Will keep for two days, covered, in fridge.

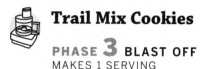

# Trail Mix Cookies

**PHASE 3 BLAST OFF**
MAKES 1 SERVING

When I can't get onto a trail for a hike, I like to bring the trail to me! These cookies are filled with all the goodies I like to pack with me on a long hike in the canyons.

**¼ cup dry almonds**

**½ teaspoon cinnamon powder**

**pinch sea salt, to taste**

**2 tablespoons walnuts**

**⅓ cup medjool dates, pitted**

**2 tablespoons raisins**

**2 tablespoons sunflower seeds**

**SUPER POWER PACK:**

**¼ teaspoon maca powder, to taste (energy enhancing)**

Combine almonds, cinnamon, and salt in food processor. Pulse into chunks. Add walnuts and pulse into chunks. Add dates, raisins, sunflower seeds, and maca, if using, and pulse to mix well. If your batter is not sticking together, add a splash of water or another medjool date to help it bind together. Or, if it's too sticky, add a bit more of the dry ingredients to get that perfect batter consistency.

Scoop about 1½ to 2 tablespoons of dough onto a sheet tray lined with parchment paper. Flatten into cookies.

Cookies will keep for several weeks or longer stored in an airtight container in the fridge, or even longer in freezer (thaw before eating).

# Watermelon Grapefruit Salad

**PHASE 3 BLAST OFF**
MAKES 2 CUPS, 1 SERVING

This is a mix of sweet fruits and savory flavors from salt, mint, and scallions and provides a new twist on the more familiar flavors of grapefruit and watermelon. Have a blast!

**1 cup grapefruit, peeled, seeded, diced, about 1 small whole**

**1 cup watermelon, diced, seeded**

**1 teaspoon scallions, sliced**

**1 teaspoon mint leaves, chiffonade**

**¼ teaspoon sea salt, to taste**

**THERMO CHARGER:**

**¼ teaspoon jalapeño pepper, seeded, minced, to taste**

Combine all ingredients, including jalapeño, if using, in a mixing bowl. Toss to mix well.

Best enjoyed immediately, but it will keep for one day, well-covered, in the fridge.

# 7

# STEADY AS SHE GOES:
# Raw Food Detox Tips +
# Maintaining Your Weight Loss

In this chapter, I'll share with you tips to help you navigate obstacles that pop up within the 15 days of the plan. After you've completed the plan, you may want to continue to incorporate more whole foods into your lifestyle, so I'll give you some ideas here for doing so easily, seamlessly, without missing a step. I'll share tips that make incorporating these healthy foods and recipes into any diet and daily routine doable, as well as how to transition to a lifestyle that includes even more raw foods. I also share some of my favorite tips on living a greener life—even how to save time, and money, prepping your food.

## SKYROCKETING TO SUCCESS

You may find yourself bumping into common stumbling blocks that often trip us up when we're trying to start out on a new path, and I want to help you avoid them. Here are some of the most common pitfalls that derail many a dieter and ideas and tips to help you manage them.

- What to do when you crave a treat
- How to navigate restaurants
- What to do during a regular workday or at office parties
- How to stay on your plan while traveling (Hint: have shake, will travel)
- What to do if a holiday lands smack dab in the middle of your detox.

## TREATING YOURSELF RIGHT

We've come to associate eating junk food and candies, ice cream, cakes, sodas with ways to "treat" ourselves. I find it interesting that the very same treats we want to wolf down the most do the most damage to our health and our collective waistlines. What gave us the idea that these were treats? How did we come to think of treating ourselves in this way as a good thing? Now, don't get me wrong here. I'm not saying one should never indulge in great tasting desserts. But I choose to eat them guilt-free, and I want you to as well. One way to do that is to use the best ingredients for optimal flavor and health. Then you can lose weight while eating dessert. And that's what we'll do on this plan.

There's nothing wrong with craving something sweet. In nature we get great vitamins, nutrients, and other good stuff in a sweet package: fruit. You can't "blow it" on this diet. To me, it's not worth taking a diet plan so seriously that massive feelings of guilt are inspired by not following it. You can make it through the 15-day plan. But you are human and there are lots of reasons, forces, and enticements that will jump into your path. I'll provide you with some delicious options that will turn cravings into weight loss weapons, not into ways to further beat up on yourself. So forget the guilt, and when you feel a craving, have one of the shakes. If that doesn't satisfy you, try one of the desserts starting on page 161.

Most importantly, remember that treating yourself right isn't only about food. It's about making choices each day that will sustain you, nourish your heart and soul, and bring some fun into your life. We've only this one time around. Why not enjoy all of it, even your diet plan? After all, at the end of the day, you're doing this for yourself. Feel great about making yourself a priority!

### 🌿 Inspiring Our Children to be Healthy

The easiest way to inspire anyone, including our kids, to be healthy, is by being a great role model of health and vitality. Kids will want to do what they see their parents doing. It's important to be active, to exercise, to play with your children. Also, when eating your treats, enjoy it very obviously. Chances are, they'll want to have a taste, too. Kids naturally gravitate to bright colors. Ever wonder why candy is colored to look like cherries, oranges, and blueberries?

## DINING OUT, TAKING OUT

I'll say it straight up: it's hard eating out if you're going to eat raw. Unless you have a local raw restaurant nearby, it can be pretty challenging. But if you want the fastest fat loss, try to keep dining out and takeout to a minimum over the next two weeks plus. Remember, it's only for 15 days. You can go back to eating out as much of whatever you choose on Day 16. But you may not want to. Why? You'll notice that as you become less padded, you're wallet will become more so, and you'll soon notice just how much money you save by not ordering in or out.

If you find that you have to dine out—say you have a business meeting or you just want to get out of the house and let someone else prepare you a meal—I've provided some guidelines that will keep you in orbit.

When I first started living this way, I used to eat before going out. Then I would enjoy a green salad and maybe a glass of wine at dinner. It could work for you, too; it certainly made it easier for me to stay away from some of the worst waist-offenders. Focus on the company, rather than on what you're eating. Don't think that you'll never be able to eat your other foods again. For a few days, you're taking a break. After you finish the plan, you can go back to eating whatever you want. Or you can explore more raw options.

Here are some more ideas for navigating the situation. It may not be pure raw, but that's okay. Keeping it as clean as possible is the way to go.

**That looks appetizing.** Order off the appetizer menu because you're likely to find salads, soups, and smaller bites there. Think volume: load up on vegetables and lean proteins. Avoid simple starches like crackers and breads, and go for whole grains instead. But try to avoid grains and starches as best you can during this program for the best results.

**Go green.** Order anything on the menu that's green and ask that it be served raw or lightly steamed, if possible. If it can only be had sautéed, ask that it be done in lemon, olive oil, garlic, and sea salt; all will add lovely flavor, without adding bad fats to the mix. Ask that a light hand be used with any oils, though.

**Have dessert at home.** This is a pretty easy one to follow, and it saves you money and unwanted calories. By the time dessert comes, you really don't have room for more food, but you dutifully stuff it down because it tastes good. Pass it up at the restaurant. Why spend the extra money, if you don't have to do so? Make one of the great recipes from this book before you go out, and enjoy the fact that your dessert will be waiting for you when you get back. You could even enjoy some dessert before you go out!

**Avoid cream sauces, deep-fried options, and other high-fat foods.** Okay, I shouldn't have to mention this in a raw food diet book, but I will because I know that temptation can be a tricky taskmaster. Instead choose dishes that are, ideally, minimally processed like fresh vegetables and fruits and legumes. If you feel you want more, order those that say poached, steamed, or baked.

**Smile at your waiter.** Perhaps one of the very best ways to navigate any restaurant situation is to be nice to your waitstaff and ask them for their help in picking the best, light choices on the menu. Let him or her know that you're trying to follow a raw diet and choose healthier foods and that you need their help in finding the best ones available at their establishment. Or, if that's not comfortable, ask them what the tastiest and healthiest thing on the menu is; they are likely to be able to reel off a number of different items. Choose what feels best to you.

**Remember your Rocket Fuels.** Look for items that include as many of the Rocket Fuel foods you're eating on the plan as possible. Ask the waiter if they can add in a few ingredients that you now know are great metabolic boosters.

**Carry on.** I've found carrying a small bottle of dressing with me makes it makes it simple to dress up a plain, big green salad, without upending my health with chemically laden processed dressings or overly fatty restaurant ones.

## WORKING IT

Okay, we all know that having a crappy day at the office is one great motivator for throwing down some junk food to feel better. Don't do it. You'll feel awful, both physically and emotionally, and you are too impor-tant to treat this badly. So what do you do instead of reaching for the pizza (or the candy dish or the cakes, pastries, and leftover sandwiches) that seem to pop up at work as soon as you start a diet? You plan ahead and you reward yourself in other ways instead.

You're shaking your head now, wondering what to do about office celebrations. The way I see it you've got two options: just go for it and enjoy the party because life is short, and it's meant to be fun, too. Or, make sure you top off your tank with good stuff before you head down the hallway to whatever event you're attending. You know you should never go to a supermarket hungry. Well, the same applies to work events. The hungrier you are, the more likely you're going to munch on things you shouldn't. Go there already satisfied, and the additional nibbles you make won't be nearly as calorically costly.

I've been known to walk around the food tables at office parties, picking off the kale décor on the edges because there were no other fresh vegetables available. Sounds weird, but it worked. I've also taken my own food to corporate off-site meetings at hotels, where lunch was catered. To be honest, after everyone else got their food and sat down to eat, what was on my plate seemed most interesting to everyone, and it would become the topic of conversation during lunch. It would actually inspire my co-workers to take better care of their health and waistlines, too! I always encourage people to lead by example.

**Have shake, will travel.** Pack your lunch and snacks and keep them nearby. If you're still hungry and you've discovered that you have four more hours at the office, remember to bring more food the next day. Volume isn't a problem on this plan; eat as much as you need of the foods I recommend. The shakes are particularly satisfying as they've been designed to provide total nutritional support. Only you will know what satiates you; so don't be afraid to eat up . . . or drink up.

**Breathe.** If you're feeling overworked, overwhelmed, or stressed, take a breather. If you can't leave your work area, then just sit there for a few moments and really focus on a few slow, long, deep breaths. They'll help to refocus you. If you can get out for a walk, even around the block or the inside hallways of your building, take it. Breath and movement are great partners in the war against stress. Studies have also shown that shorter bursts of activity, like 10 minutes, several times a day, have health benefits. So you don't always have to work out in 30-minute chunks; it can be less, and it does make a difference.

**Talk it out.** If you just can't get your head off the brownies down the hall, grab a friend and chat for a few minutes. Or grab the phone during your break and call someone you love. Better yet, if you have a detox partner, reach out for support and to check in to see how she or he is doing with the plan. More often than not, just taking those moments to connect to someone else will give you what you need to squash your craving. Sometimes, we all just need a little redirection, and a good friend can be the best distraction.

Of course, doing this program with a friend can be both fun and helpful. Having someone to support you throughout the next 15 days is invaluable. You'll be more likely to succeed with a little friendly competition going.

**Bring dessert.** If you want to reap the full benefit of the Blast-Off plan, you'll want to take your own desserts to whatever event is going on that day. Bring some of my slimming, beautifying recipes and enjoy them with a smile. Desserts taste better without guilt. Remember, you're allowed to share, and you'll be spreading good health and great taste along the way. I recommend taking the Peach Crumble (page 163) and/or Fudge Brownie with Fresh Berries (page 161); they'll be a big hit. I guarantee it.

I take desserts to events and potlucks, place them on the table with all the other food, and don't even mention that they are healthy or raw, and no one even guesses they are. Do this test and see for yourself how much others will enjoy them because good food is good food, and they are delicious, hands down. This is actually where my catering business and SmartMonkey Foods® began, with people asking me to bring my raw recipes, especially desserts, with me to events because they were so yummy!

## ON THE ROAD AGAIN

If you've ever taken a road trip, you know that traveling our nation's highways is not conducive to eating healthful, nourishing foods. And if you still actually get food on airplanes, the same would be true there. So what can you do? Again, it's all in the planning.

And guess what? This is where eating foods closest to their natural state is actually going to be a great benefit. If you choose the right ones, many of our Rocket Fuels come perfectly packaged. Clean 'em off and eat 'em up! You won't have to worry about lugging your meals around in coolers or finding somewhere to heat them in a microwave. They come perfectly packaged.

**Check it out before you check in.** Before you depart on your trip, search online for farmers' markets or natural food stores near your hotel. What I like to do is to check in and drop off my bags at the hotel. Then I immediately venture out for fruits, vegetables, and water to stock my room. If my hotel room doesn't have a fridge, I'll buy items that keep well at room temperature like lemon for my water and salads, apples, bananas, carrots, cucumbers, raw nuts and seeds, nut butter, dried fruits, and kefir or kombucha for probiotics. I know I need extra immune-boosting 'Bots, especially when traveling.

**Go nuts!** Stock up on pistachios, almonds, and walnuts and have a handful with each meal. (Of course, remember that raw, unsalted nuts are the way to go.) Toss them on a salad. Or enjoy them as snacks. Pistachios are the leanest of them, so if you're concerned about overdoing it on the calories, feel free to enjoy these beauties pretty freely. They travel well, don't take up much room in luggage, and don't require refrigeration. I like to make up my own trail mix with nuts, seeds, goji berries, golden berries, and cacao nibs, and carry them in a small glass jar.

**Go Hefty.** I'm joking a little bit about this, but bring a huge bag of lettuces (yes, you'll have to wash, tear and dry in advance, but it will be worth it) along on your trip. Chop up some peppers, radishes, carrots, celery; bring some cherry or grape tomatoes; in general, grab as many bite-size veggies as you can and throw them into your big bag. Or re-use the grocery bags you get at your local market and bring a few along. If you've carefully dried all the vegetables before placing them in the bag(s) (and you put a few paper towels in there as well), dressing-free they should keep nicely in a cooler. Don't store the cooler in the sun; choose a dark, cool place. Then freely enjoy salads whenever you need to stop for a rest break.

If you're not traveling with a cooler, lettuces won't fare so well. Personally, I gravitate toward heartier greens like kales, chards, and veggies that can stay out of the cooler for a bit like jicima, carrot, and celery. In a cooler, of course, they all keep longer.

**Veg out.** I travel with cucumbers, carrots, apples, avocados, nori sheets, chlorella tablets, celery, radishes, and lemon (to use as dressing or put in my water). There's no need for refrigeration with any of these choices, so they'll be fine for a day or two, or longer at room temperature. Plus, sea vegetables take up very little space and are light to carry. A big pack of nori sheets fits perfectly into the outside pocket of my carry-on luggage. And wakame hydrates and grows three to four times its size in water.

**Go to a bar.** Snack bar, that is. If you need something quick and fast, and you can't stand another salad (hey, it happens), then grab a snack bar. I've provided you with a couple of recipes in the following chapter; plus the Trail Mix Cookies and Brownie recipes work great as bars, too. So pop a few in your purse or briefcase. If you run out or don't feel like making them, there are few decent, commercially made bars. Just make sure you can read all the ingredients in the bar you choose to buy. Ideally, it will include whole fruits, nuts, and seeds, with no chemical preservatives or flavorings, and no added refined sugars.

**Get juiced.** Find a local juice bar, if you can, and ask the staff to prepare you a fresh drink. Go for veggies, first. If they only have fruit drink options, be sure you specify that you don't want any sugar or syrup added to your drink, just water and fruit. Some establishments make their drinks taste "better" by adding sugars and syrups to the mix; be a savvy consumer and you'll be able to avoid this.

**You can take it with you.** When traveling to spots where healthy food options are a challenge, I carry a small blender in my luggage. It's about the size of a small pair of shoes. This makes it easy to blend fruits and vegetables with my own Rocket Fuel powders like dehydrated alfalfa grass, hemp protein, flax meal, and spirulina to make my perfect shakes. I love travel blenders because they come with lids that make it easy to take your shake with you and drink it from the same container you blended it in.

## HOLIDAY . . . CELEBRATE

Okay, you've bought this book and are ready to start the plan, but "name your holiday" is just around the corner. What should you do? You've numerous options. Personally, I'd say why start the plan now so that right smack in the middle of it you'll be tempted by every goodie known to man? Or, you could go with the plan for whatever days you can, enjoy your holiday, then get back on it right after. You won't see the same weight-loss benefit, but that's okay, too, because you'll have "book ended" any health-harming activities with lots of fresh, wholesome foods. There's a third and fourth option, too: you could do the plan before the holiday or save it for afterward. I've said it before. It's your life. Your plan. Your choice.

I am being a little sneaky here because I know that once you start eating this way, you'll feel so much better, your energy levels will sky rocket, and your skin will glow. So it doesn't matter to me when you start, as long as you do, because you'll get hooked on the results! Follow your needs and your gut. Join me on the diet when you can.

If you decide to stay on this plan during holidays and special events, the same tips apply as eating out and navigating office parties. I'm known to follow this plan especially during the holidays because I get a double bonus that way. Not only do I clean out my engines, fill up my tank with nutritious, clean food, and blast unwanted pounds, I also avoid doing damage to my body and adding on extra pounds I'll only have to shed later.

**Don't be a party pooper.** Fill up before going out to the party. Enjoy a shake or full meal, so you can focus on connecting with the people at the party, rather than on what to eat there. It should always be more about the company than the food anyway, right?

**Share.** Ask if you can bring a dish to share. Again, I think my raw food desserts are a gateway food for inspiring others to consider taking better care of their health. They slide in under the radar, undetected, as yummy food. It's that simple.

**Bring snacks.** Trail mix, nuts, energy bars all fit in your pocket or purse, and they're easy to reach for and pop into your mouth without drawing much attention to what you're eating, or rather, what you're not eating.

**Just say no.** Sometimes a host or hostess or others you're celebrating with may feel uncomfortable if you're not participating by eating the food they are eating. I like to avoid drawing attention to myself, what I'm eating, or what I'm not eating. But if pressed, you can just say you're trying a new way of eating, or a new diet plan, and though you'd love to enjoy what they are sharing/eating, you politely have to beg off for now. Sometimes, when the host is super persistent, I'll make up some other excuse like having food allergies, or that I ate something bad and my belly hasn't been feeling well. No one can argue with you when you're not feeling well, right?

## NOW WHAT? MAINTAINING YOUR WEIGHT LOSS

Now that you've let go of excess fat, cleaned up your body, and are super-charged with nutrients, I know you feel fantastic. If you're like me, you're going to want to hold onto that radiance, that glow. So I'll give you some tips on how to maintain it.

You've watched the pounds Shake It Up, Melt Down, and then Blast Off. Perhaps you've reached your goal weight, and you feel great and you look awesome. So what's next? How much further do you want to go? Want to try another week? Month? Or do you want to learn how to incorporate more of this food and the healthy shakes into your normal routine? Here are tips and tricks for blasting through to the next level of your health goal.

## IF YOU NEED TO SHED MORE

If you have more weight to lose, I recommend repeating Phases 1 and 2 once or twice in sequence, then moving on to Phase 3. You can stay on Phase 3 quite easily for as long as you feel is needed. Or you can choose to repeat all three phases until you reach your goal. If you don't want or need a detox, you could also stay on Phases 2 and 3 until you are where you want to be. This is your plan. Use it as it suits your busy lifestyle.

My general rule for continued weight loss, as long as you have excess fat to lose, is to always enjoy shakes for breakfast and snacks. Let the blender help you, so it's easier for your body to absorb all the nutrients to power pack your body. Enjoy salad for lunch, and do your best to skip the carbs from bread and croutons. Add protein from seeds or nuts, or if you choose animal protein, pick lower toxin options like free-range organic chicken, beef, bison, or wild, low-mercury fish. Enjoy a raw food meal for dinner, even if paired with animal protein like organic turkey or bison. Skip the bread and pasta, excess sugar, and carbs, which your body will store as fat, especially later in the day or evening.

## ☆ If You Can't Go All the Way Raw

Here are some other rich sources of Rocket Fuels:

### Probiotics:
- Buttermilk
- Yogurt
- Soft cheeses
- Tempeh

### Prebiotics:
- Legumes
- Tomatoes
- Wheat

### MCFAs, Omega 3s, and MUFAs:
These animal sources of the various fat-blasting fatty acids are not part of the 15-day plan, but if you later choose to incorporate them into your lifestyle, I believe it's important you know about the food you are eating—even if it's not the food I'd advocate. And, with fish, beware of mercury levels and polluted waters! Check out Monterey Bay Aquarium's Seafood Watch program

for recommended low mercury and sustainable choices:
http://www.montereybayaquarium.org/cr/seafoodwatch.aspx

- Organic butter or cream
- Organic chicken
- Shrimp (low mercury, eat no more than 12 ounces per week)
- Halibut (moderate mercury, eat no more than 4 ounces a week)
- Snapper (moderate mercury, eat no more than 4 ounces a week)

The best choices contain the lowest levels of mercury and are highest in healthy fats:

- Wild Salmon
- Mackerel (Atlantic, jack, chub)
- Sardines
- Halibut

This plan has been presented to you as a diet, but in reality, it's a lifestyle. There are people who thrive by following a diet like Phase 2, but even more people maintain a long-term eating style that's very like Phase 3. It's easy to incorporate the fundamental principles of this plan into your way of approaching eating and life. I basically live Phase 3 all the time. When I've been traveling and eating less than optimal foods and have fallen off my routine, I like to use Phase 1 to reboot myself before returning to my regular lifestyle. Otherwise, Phase 3 is for me.

## HAVING A BLAST—
## LIVING THE LIFESTYLE ON YOUR OWN TERMS

After 15 days of shakes, you're now a pro at whipping up delicious nutrient blasters in your blender. Perhaps you've gotten into the habit of starting off your days with a shake. This is a great habit to continue with, forever. I like to start my days with nutrient-rich shakes because they, along with green vegetable juice, act as my personal daily multi-vitamin. It's an amazing way to jumpstart your engine each and every morning.

The snacks you've learned to make during the past 15 days all work wonderfully as snacks beyond this diet plan. So when you're hungry and ready to reach for a healthy snack, make it one from the 15-Day Raw Food Detox.

All the recipes from this plan make great additions to any type of meal. Each of the dishes you learned to make pair perfectly with a piece of wild caught, low mercury fish; organic, antibiotic-free, grass-fed, free-range chicken, turkey, or beef; bison; as well as vegetarian and vegan proteins like quinoa, legumes, tofu, and tempeh. (My favorite is quinoa. It's an amino-acid-rich protein that's easy to find at natural food stores. I like to scoop it onto my salads and add it to my wraps.)

You already started menu planning by putting together your own Day 15 meals based on your favorites from this book. Now that you've finished your diet and are on to the rest of your life, you can choose to try out and include in your lifestyle plan any of the recipes from my previous books: *Ani's Raw Food Kitchen, Ani's Raw Food Desserts, Ani's Raw Food Essentials,* and *Ani's Raw Food Asia.*

 **Happiness**

Choosing to eat clean, whole, fresh, and raw foods is more than just a diet. It's a lifestyle that helps us be kinder to the planet while helping us look and feel our best. When we feel great, it's easy to be happy.

Here are some daily happiness tips to consider:

■ Forgive

■ Be compassionate

■ Make amends

■ Be generous

■ Be kind

■ Strive for inner peace and happiness

■ Make a positive difference in the world

■ Be hope-filled

■ Oh, and remember to turn off the TV.

Remember to choose whole foods straight from Mother Earth, and do your best to avoid foods created in a factory like fake soy meats, soy yogurts, fake cheeses, and other popular vegan junk foods. Those foods are processed and contain hidden ingredients that make you fat, like GMOs, MSG, sodium, unhealthy fats, and high fructose corn syrup.

The next time you're making dinner for a party or a special guest, start the meal with your favorite soup, then move on to a snack for an appetizer, a main dish paired with a lean protein, and blow the top off the meal with a delicious dessert. All of my cookbooks have great recipes to choose from. You'll help rev up your guests' engines with all the fresh flavors, colors, aromas, and nutrients. And they'll thank you for making them feel great.

## MAKING THE LEAP:
## TRANSITIONING TO A HIGH RAW LIFESTYLE

Health is a lifelong pursuit; it doesn't just happen overnight. This journey is about doing the best we can each day and in each moment. By noticing how great we feel, how much better we feel than we did the previous day, and striving to feel just as good or better the next day, we create our wellness one step at a time. Health is a continuum, where we move from one end of the spectrum slowly over to the opposite end, toward ultimate vigor and longevity.

My approach to incorporating more whole, clean, fresh, healthy foods into any diet is not one of deprivation. Rather, I choose to include more and more of those good-for-us ingredients and recipes like the shakes, green salads, and desserts we've been making the past 15 days with any meal. Start by enjoying these first, and they'll fill you up with their fiber, water, and rich nutrients to satisfy you. Then, move on to the rest of your meal. Soon, you'll notice that you have less room and desire for the least beneficial foods on your table, and you will naturally eat less of them. Over time, what I've seen happen repeatedly is that folks automatically shift toward a cleaner, healthier, whole-food diet, without much effort at all, and without deprivation. Here are a few more ideas for keeping you steady on the path to lifelong health.

**Start with raw food first.** Add on a shake, a large green salad, and/or dessert to your meal and enjoy these first. Like I explained earlier, these fiber-, water-, and nutrient-rich foods will fill you up before you even start eating the rest of your meal. You'll eat less of the other stuff, but you won't feel deprived because you're allowed to eat it but just won't want to because your belly's already full. This inclusion of healthy, clean, fresh foods naturally elbows out the less than healthy foods for an easy transition to a healthier diet and lifestyle.

**Take note.** Start by noticing how you feel at the beginning, during, and at the end of each day. (I started you on this habit with the questions at the end of each day's menu plan.) You may notice how light and vibrant you feel, how energized you are, how clear your mind is, how radiant your skin looks, how happy you are to feel good. Sometimes we really don't realize that we weren't feeling great until we experience what it's like to really feel good. Once we can recognize the difference, it makes it easy to strive to do better and better each day. Now that we feel great, it's harder to choose to feel bad.

**How fresh are you?** With each new day, decide how much fresh, whole, healthy, clean food you'd like to add to your diet. Perhaps you'd like to add in a shake with all your meals, plus a green salad at lunch and dinner. This will help fill you up and keep you satisfied. Desserts are easy to add to any meal, or even to enjoy as a meal or snack all on their own. Unlike baked desserts, raw food desserts are made from nuts, seeds, and fruit—all whole foods, fresh, and nutritious. Again, there's no guilt here, which is a dream come true for me!

**Double down.** When making recipes, double or triple up the batches and keep leftovers in the fridge. This way you have fast, easy-to-grab, healthy snacks always at the ready. Just like we keep a carton of dairy milk or bottle of dressing in the fridge, it helps to keep raw versions of these items on hand in the same way. What I love about making multiple batches at once is that your set up, prep, and clean up don't take much more time or work than when making just a single batch.

**Gratitude.** Now, on the days where we may not adhere as strictly to our goals or plan, we definitely want to avoid adding additional stress or guilt onto ourselves. You know about cortisol by now, the stress hormone, and how it makes us store belly fat. Instead of stressing, choose appreciation and gratitude. We're blessed to be living the lives we live.

I live in California, where we grow food to feed the rest of the country. I'm lucky to have the option to decline food because it may not be organic or vegan, for example, when so many other people are starving on our planet. I have hot running water, a shower, and a flushing toilet. Gratitude and appreciation help me to keep things in perspective.

**Only you.** You're the only one who really ever knows what you need, what will work best for your lifestyle, for your mind, body, and spirit. What works for someone else, won't necessarily work for you. I recommend reading as many books as possible and listening to lectures and talks to learn what's worked for others, and then pick and choose what you'd like to test on yourself. See how each works for you. Ultimately, you'll want to create a personalized lifestyle that works just for you, and that will change over time as you do.

When I first shifted over to my gourmet raw food diet and lifestyle, I stuffed myself full of complex recipes with lots of natural sugar from fruits and healthy fats from nuts and seeds. That was over 15 years ago, and today, I eat mostly greens, sea vegetables, and protein, and keep my fat and sugar levels in check. The foods I eat have become less complex, and my personal recipes use only a couple ingredients, instead of 20 or 30. I still enjoy more complex, gourmet recipes, but only on occasion. Follow your own tastes and needs; if you're reaching for health, they won't steer you wrong.

**Make it hard to fail.** Keep healthier raw food snacks on hand to make it easy to grab them for a quick snack. Keep Trail Mix Cookies, Fudge Brownies, Cobbler Crumble, shakes, soups, and mylks around, just as you would the cooked varieties.

**Gather recipes.** I keep a notebook in the kitchen, and I write down every recipe I make with notes on what worked and what didn't. Try it out. Don't forget the 5-star rating system from the menu plans either. It will make it easier for you, like it does for me, to find recipes you like that you can choose from when trying to figure out what to make.

**Mix it up.** Eat a mix of different foods. Always try your best to choose organic, local, and seasonal foods when possible. But it's also very important to eat different varieties and types of fresh, whole foods. Each food has its own unique nutritional profile and its own special flavor and combination of health benefits. Don't get stuck eating the same thing over and over. This is where CSA, or community supported agriculture, is amazing. By pre-paying a farmer for a box of weekly fruits and vegetables, you'll get whatever's ripe and ready that week in your box, including items you may normally not think to buy.

## GOING CLEAN WITHOUT SPENDING TOO MUCH GREEN

How do we put a price on our health? I spend most of my money on the highest quality organic foods I can get my hands on, and I don't even think twice about it. I've learned to make my health and happiness my first priority because when I feel great, anything in life is possible. Plus, I'm avoiding health care costs in the future by staying healthy today. I don't like to acquire many physical possessions, and I live simply, even though I do love luxury goods and fashion. I choose to buy most of my items secondhand because it saves me a ton of money, and it's another way to tread lightly on Mother Earth. Here are some money-saving eco tips for finding healthy ingredients for less.

**Bulk up.** Buying in bulk means spending more of our money on the actual food, not the packaging, stickers, and manufacturing. Shopping locally at farmers' markets means you can buy in bulk, while also avoiding paying for the distributing, marketing, and storing of factory-processed foods. Do this and you're actually getting more food for your money. As I mentioned previously, you can also look for supermarkets' weekly sale items and, if you have time, shop across multiple stores for sale items.

**Put a lid on it.** Freeze ripe fruit for shakes or dehydrate it to preserve it. Buy sale vegetables and pickle them so they last longer. Remember, pickles are full of our friends the 'Bots that eat our belly fat and boost our immune system. You can find many pickled vegetable recipes in *Ani's Raw Food Essentials* and *Ani's Raw Food Asia*.

**Grow wild.** Plant a garden and grow your own veggies and fruits. Better yet, learn how to forage for wild edibles. Food that grows in the wild are so strong they don't need to be sprayed for pests or watered to grow. That's powerful.

**Do it again.** Save money and resources by reusing bags, jars, containers, and anything else you can find a second use for. Don't purchase new storage containers or anything else that you can get for free when buying any type of packaged good. Also, buy books and kitchen equipment secondhand.

## SAVING TIME IN THE KITCHEN

I just shared ways to keep food costs lower, more eco-nomical™. Well, as you know from this book, healthy food doesn't have to take all day to prepare either. Here are more ideas for living clean and raw without living in the kitchen.

**Batch it.** You've seen me say this a few times now in the book, but this one bears repeating: make multiple batches when preparing your recipes. Making multiple batches at once doesn't take more total time or much more energy than making a single batch.

**Stock up on staples.** Keep ingredient staples on hand like nuts, seeds, herbs, spices, so it's easy to whip up a snack any time. Also keep a few raw food basics in your pantry like dressings, sauces, mylk, and desserts. Other staples include rawnola, buckwheat crispies, crackers, breads, biscuits, cookies, kale chips, for which you'll find recipes in my prior books, especially *Ani's Raw Food Essentials*.

**Make, store, and pour.** Make and store your foods in the same container. For example, blend your sauce or dressing using your personal blender. Store it by using the container's screw top lid to close the container, and keep it in the fridge for a longer shelf-life. This means fewer items to clean up and less water wasted doing so.

**Keep it clean.** Organize your fridge; make it neat and orderly (see my tips on doing this on page 53). Keep your countertop work area clean and tidy, with all your dry ingredients nearby but clearly labeled and organized logically. This makes it simple to grab the ingredient you need to whip up a healthy treat.

**Set the stage.** In a commercial kitchen, *mise en place* means having ingredients organized, arranged, in place, and ready to be used to help the chef avoid stopping and assembling items while cooking, which speeds up food prep. Before you start, set out the equipment you'll be using and all the ingredients you'll need to make your recipe. Place each ingredient, pre-measured into a small container or bowl, so it's ready to go. This way, you'll be able to make your recipe in a snap! It also will help ensure you have everything you need, right up front.

**Prewash.** Before I begin a recipe, I wash all my ingredients. This way, I avoid stopping midway to clean my produce.

**Get scrappy.** I put a big container on my counter to catch all my compost: the scraps like peelings, shavings, stems, or ends of carrots and squash. This saves me from having to run back and forth to and from the garbage can and makes composting easier, too, if you're of the mind or have the space to do so. Kanga, my dog, makes for a wonderful compost bin. I process these scraps with nuts, seeds, sea vegetables, and coconut or olive oil to make her a Kanga Paté that she loves. (Look for "Kanga's Dandy Dog Food" chapter, in *Ani's Raw Food Kitchen*.)

Now that we've streamlined your body—and your kitchen and prep time—next on the flight schedule is how to reach for health goals that go beyond weight loss and keep you flying straight and into the Next Stage.

# PART 3

# THE REST
# OF THE STORY

# 8

# THE NEXT STAGE

Now that you've blasted and kept off the pounds and you feel great, maybe you're interested in exploring new terrains? That's what this chapter is all about: taking your health to a whole new level and fine-tuning what you've learned so as to maximize the performance of your body. I've divided the chapter into three mini plans: enhancing endurance, building muscle and strength, and improving flexibility. I'll also offer up a few tips for immune-proofing your body.

You've cleaned your engine, tanked it up with great Rocket Fuels, made it lean and sleek, and now you can choose which area you want to supercharge even more.

Want to train for a marathon? Or just want to chase a few little kids around all day? Well, you'll need to have amazing endurance in either case. The foods, tips, and recipes in this chapter can give you that. Want to build even more muscle now that you've shed the excess fat? I'll show you how to move and what to eat to accomplish that. Feel like you've been getting a little "creaky" and not at your limber best? Want to take your sport to the next level? You can become more flexible (all of us can), and it will enhance your body's ability to move with grace and ease.

It's all here. Everything you need to build the best you. These small bites are designed to go down easily and have you living, eating, and *un*cooking your way to optimal health all year long.

## MAXIMIZING ENDURANCE AND ENERGY

### PUT THE KEY IN THE IGNITION:
WHAT YOU NEED FOR OPTIMAL ENERGY

Our bodies use energy all the time; every single function requires it. By now, following Blast Off, you should be feeling pretty revved up. The plan you've been adhering to is carefully crafted to give you abundant energy. But there are times, like when training for an athletic event or when your life hits a particularly rough patch, that you need a little extra boost. Here are some valuable tips and reminders for sailing through these moments.

- Pair Sugars with Fats
- Don't Forget Green Tea or Cacao
- Make Room for Maca
- Get Your ZZZZs
- Get Your Os—Omega 3s
- Get Your Bs—B Vitamins
- Amp Up Antioxidants
- Jettison Stressors
- Live Clean and Green

### PAIR SUGARS WITH FATS,
### 20 MINUTES BEFORE EXERCISE

Eat higher sugar, higher calorie fruits (dates, bananas, plums, pears, pineapple, orange, mango) with a fat source (nuts, seeds, or nut butters, coconut oil, or coconut milk) for longer, sustained energy. Try to eat these sugars 20 minutes prior to a workout for longer performance. Also, if you want energy levels that soar you have to continue to avoid highly refined carbohydrates; instead choose to eat the right carbs and fats as your main fuel source. No, a candy bar with raisins won't fit the bill here. Got it? Also, don't forget to fill up on fiber for more sustained energy levels throughout each day. Fiber is what time-releases sugar into the bloodstream. You won't have a spiked sugar high and then crash later.

## DON'T FORGET THE GREEN TEA OR CACAO

Not only are both good for all the reasons listed prior, but the caffeine inside of both is a known physical performance booster. But one caveat: You don't want to overdo it on caffeinated beverages and foods. If you reach too often for them, you could end up right back where you started . . . more fatigued from blowing out your adrenals. As with everything in life, it's all about balance. One serving each of green tea and cacao a day, and you should be good to go.

## MAKE ROOM FOR MACA

By now you know that maca is one of my favorite foods. With a high protein content (important for training) and a wide variety of amino acids (20 of them), it's high in calcium and B vitamins, contains sterols (good for bodybuilders), and is packed with healthy fatty acids. It's not a stimulant; with the green tea and cacao, you've enough of those in your system. It's a great choice for increasing energy, stamina, and endurance. It's known as an adaptogen, which means it strengthens our ability to handle stress. It makes us stronger and rebuilds our adrenals. That's why I like to couple maca with caffeine; maca offsets any adrenal stress that could come from too much caffeine.

## GET YOUR ZZZZs

You have likely heard over and over again how important it is to get enough sleep. It helps keep you healthy, slender, and, yes, energized. Yet way too many of us don't get enough of it. We go to bed too late, needing just a few more moments to ourselves at the end of the workday. We get up too early, needing to prepare lunch for the kids or finish a last-minute project. When we lack sleep and our stress levels are high, our cortisol levels increase, which makes us store belly fat. That's exactly what we don't want to be doing!

I get it. I've been there myself. But very few of us function at our prime when we don't take the time to snuggle down, rest, and recharge. Sleep at least six hours each night; seven to eight is optimal. I love when I get to sleep eight or nine hours; it's such a treat, and I wake feeling great and powerful! If you're restless or suffering insomnia, try meditating or doing some calming yoga moves before bed. I've had my struggles with insomnia, and I found that even meditating in bed rather than worrying about not being able to sleep helps. Hot lavender oil baths help, too. It all starts, though, with making sure you put sleep at the top of your priority list. Sleep's at the top of the list for me, even if it means missing a party or social engagement. I find when I go to bed at 10 p.m. or 11 p.m., I get the best rest. It's the most important thing you need "to do" today and every day. Get into bed at a reasonable time, and the rest will follow.

## GET YOUR Os—OMEGA 3s

I'm not going to boast about Omega 3s again, so this will be short (if you want a refresher, you can always go back to the beginning of the book and review the basic Rocket Fuels). But you need these healthy fats for their calories (more healthy calories = more energy). Don't forget to reach for them whenever you need a charge. And women, don't be afraid of these fats; the female body during exercise primarily reaches for fat for fuel, while men rely more heavily on protein.

*Top Your Tank: Flaxseed, walnuts, soybeans (cooked), and tofu (cooked).*

## GET YOUR Bs

If you want to increase endurance, particularly if you're training for a 5K race or anything else that you need more energy for, you must make sure you are getting enough B vitamins, as well as glutamine, CoQ10, magnesium, sulfur, and iron. All of these nutrients are major players in energy production in the human body. Athletes tend to use more iron, as well as need more glutamine and magnesium. Anyone who has ever suffered from iron-deficiency anemia knows just how weak and fatigued it can leave you.

Glutamine, found in plant sources like raw spinach, raw parsley, cabbage, beets, and beans (cooked), as well as animal products like meat and dairy, is important to counteract muscle breakdown and to immune system function. Our body produces enough glutamine to meet our needs, so supplementation is usually unnecessary, unless perhaps you're under extremely high levels of stress. Cortisol, the "stress hormone," can lower glutamine levels. Glutamine supports a healthy immune system and helps to remove ammonia from the body.

Magnesium plays a pivotal role in ATP production. Think of ATP, adenosine triphosphate, as your personal cellular ATM energy bank; it allows you access to your energy. CoQ10 is necessary to mitochondrial performance (mitochondria are like little energy "factories" in your cells).
*Top Your Tank: Almonds, brazil nuts, broccoli, brussels sprouts, cabbage, kale, leafy greens, parsley, pumpkin seeds, quinoa, sesame seeds, spinach, sprouted whole grains, and sunflower seeds. When choosing sprouted whole grains, it's best to go for the actual raw sprouts. You can find them baked into breads as well. But they are best raw, fresh, unprocessed with no milling, canning, or preserving.*

## AMP UP ANTIOXIDANTS—A, C, E, AND SELENIUM

The more energy a body produces, the more byproducts (free radicals) of that energy also get produced in the bloodstream. These byproducts are like garbage that gets put on the curb or street corner; they need to be cleaned up for your streets/blood vessels to be kept safe and for the rest of your property to remain intact. And the best guys for the job of cleaning up free radicals are the protective antioxidants or ACES: vitamin A/beta carotene, vitamin C, vitamin E, and selenium.
*Top Your Tank: Almonds, bell peppers, Brazil nuts, broccoli, cantaloupe, carrots, cayenne, chili powder, citrus fruits, papaya, paprika, pine nuts, sweet potatoes, squash (cooked), strawberries, and sunflower seeds.*

## JETTISON STRESSORS

This is a tricky one, isn't it? We're all surrounded on all sides each day with multiple things that can kick up a stress tornado at any time. Try to take it easy on yourself; be kind to yourself. And the best way to do it is to clear the decks. Take a look at all the key areas of your life—house, work, family—and really think about ways you can chill out more in each arena. Pick one thing to address each week; it can be small or big, but it has to be something that's adding to your stress load. And if you can't get rid of it (most of us can't afford to fire our jobs/bosses or kids), see what you can do to minimize the power it has over your life. If the stress is something deeper—the loss of a loved one or an illness—the result is the same: you need to increase joy and decrease the burden you're carrying. Eating right, sleeping well, and taking care of yourself are all keys to doing so.

Here are a few foods that contain calming folate and B vitamins. They can help you a bit as you jettison some of the energy drains adversely affecting your life.

***Top Your Tank:*** *Arugula, basil, maca, quinoa, and sunflower seeds.*

## LIVE CLEAN AND GREEN

I can't leave this section without stressing that it's not just choosing the wrong foods that can be toxic to us and our vibrancy. You must also take the time and care to decrease ancillary toxins in your environment, if for no other reason than that your cells perform better if they, too, are cleaner. Better cell function = more energy.

The Environmental Protection Agency says indoor air can be two to five times more polluted than outdoor air, even in the largest and most industrialized cities. So be aware of poisons that enter your environment via the air you breathe (outgassing from paint on your walls, carpet, and fabric on your furniture, and toxic cleaning products that sit under your bathroom sink) and from chemicals that are absorbed through your skin (beauty products and clothing fabric).

☆ **Was Popeye Wrong?**

The iron in plant food may be harder for your body to absorb than the iron in meat. So where does that leave those of us who want to eat non-animal foods? In good shape, actually. Researchers uncovered that eating vitamin C-rich foods can triple, even quadruple, the amount of iron you get from your food. So pair up spinach and peppers, broccoli and pumpkin seeds, strawberries and pecans— you get the picture.

## EATING FOR ENDURANCE: THE RECIPES

Enjoying these recipes will definitely bump up your game. Each works wonderfully on it's own for pre- and post-workout and can easily be paired with a raw meal. Dense animal protein may actually weigh you down pre-workout, but these recipes make great sides and accompaniments to all types of meals, even paired with organic grass-fed chicken, bison, or wild-caught, low-mercury fish. Feel free to use these recipes however you see fit.

 ### Banana, Spinach, Chocolate Power Smoothie

**PHASES 2 AND 3 BREAKFAST OR SNACK**
MAKES 2 SERVINGS

The carbohydrates in a banana are from three sugars: fructose, sucrose, and glucose. Combined with fiber, they give us both instant and sustained energy. Fuel up with two bananas for a long workout because they digest more slowly than most fruit. The recipe gives you additional protein power from almonds, spirulina, and spinach, with a rocket boost from raw cacao powder.

> 2 cups bananas, from about 2 whole
>
> 1 cup spinach leaves, washed well
>
> ¼ cup almond butter, raw
>
> 1 tablespoon cacao powder
>
> 1 teaspoon spirulina powder
>
> 3 cups Thai baby coconut water, or filtered water
>
> 1 cup ice, optional

Place all ingredients, except ice, into a high-speed blender. Blend until smooth. Add ice, if using, and blend to mix well. Enjoy immediately.

Will keep for one day, sealed tightly, in the fridge.

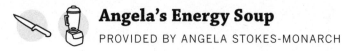

## Angela's Energy Soup

PROVIDED BY ANGELA STOKES-MONARCH

**PHASES 2 AND 3** LUNCH, DINNER, OR SNACK
MAKES 1 SERVING

Use your blender to whip up a quick, tasty soup that travels well and is packed with nutrifying ingredients.

**1/2 cucumber, chopped**

**1/2 red or yellow bell pepper, chopped**

**1 generous handful of leafy greens: spinach, kale, lettuce, etc.**

**1 little bunch coriander**

**1 clove garlic**

**juice of half a lemon**

**1 little handful dulse**

**either 3 tablespoons tahini or the flesh of a small avocado**

**filtered water—maybe 3 cups—so that its reaches about half way up the blender, once all the veggies are inside**

Place everything into a high-speed blender, blend, and serve. Angela usually stirs in some coconut chips or even mung bean sprouts to chew on.

##  Philip's Spinach Bisque Soup

COURTESY OF PHILIP MCCLUSKEY

**PHASE 3** LUNCH, DINNER, OR SNACK
MAKES 1 SERVING

Philip says he created the base of this creamy spinach soup to be reminiscent of heavy cream, but it uses heart-healthy macadamia nuts or hemp seed instead. A touch of nutmeg, cumin, and chili adds warming, fragrant spices.

**1 cup spinach**

**¼ cup raw macadamia nuts (or 2 tablespoons hemp butter)**

**1 tablespoon nutritional yeast**

**1 tablespoon miso, any color**

¼ teaspoon garlic, peeled and chopped

1 teaspoon cumin

⅛ to ¼ teaspoon chili powder, to taste

1/2 teaspoon freshly grated nutmeg (or powdered nutmeg)

sea salt and freshly ground pepper, to taste

2 cups filtered water

Blend all ingredients together in the high-speed blender until smooth.

Add salt and pepper to taste and serve with a touch of nutritional yeast and/or chili powder.

 ## Goji Chia Energy Cereal

PHASE **3** BREAKFAST OR SNACK
MAKES 2 SERVINGS

Aztec warriors used chia as a high-energy food on their conquests. One tablespoon of chia seeds is said to provide lasting energy, stamina, and endurance for 24 hours. Chia is loaded with Omega-3 fatty acids and is said to have the highest antioxidant activity of any whole food. Just 2 tablespoons of chia seed added to your daily diet adds about 7 grams fiber, 2 grams protein, 205 milligrams calcium, and 5 grams Omega 3s. Enjoy this cereal with a blended nut mylk that's super easy to make with nuts and water, or you can always use your favorite almond or rice milk if you don't have a blender handy.

### MYLK

¼ cup nuts, raw, any type like Brazil, cashew, almond

2 cups filtered water

### CEREAL

¼ cup chia seeds

¼ cup goji berries

1 tablespoon maca powder, optional

Blend mylk by placing nuts and water into a high-speed blender. Blend until smooth, and then set aside. Place chia, goji, and maca, if using, into a large soup or cereal bowl. Add 2 cups mylk, and stir to mix well. Set aside for 15 to 30 minutes, stirring a few times to ensure seeds are hydrating evenly.

**Variations:** Try mixing in additional ingredients to your basic Goji Chia Energy Cereal before serving like 1 tablespoon cacao powder and/or nibs, 2 tablespoons carob powder, 1 tablespoon alcohol-free vanilla extract, crushed nuts, and/or a dash of stevia to sweeten.

## START YOUR ENGINES: THE ENERGY WORKOUT

You can't be healthy if you don't move. Period. If you're coming to this section for tips, you likely already know that and are here to supercharge it. To help build endurance, you need to increase your functional strength, and the aim is to build strength without adding bulk. This will help your muscles perform more efficiently. Interval training, like jogging between street lights, then sprinting to the next street light, then jogging between, then sprinting again will help build stamina and endurance quickly, and help strengthen your muscles for longer distance running. Between interval days, go longer distances, what we call LSD for long slow distance, once or twice a week.

My friend, professional athlete, champion mountain runner, and stair climbing champion Tim Van Orden turned me on to Tabata interval training. The Tabata Protocol is a high-intensity workout program wherein you warm up for 5 minutes, do eight intervals of 20 seconds of high-intensity exercise or sprints, followed by 10 seconds of rest, followed by a 2-minute cool down.

There's a huge field two blocks from my home, and I jog there to warm up; then I sprint 20 seconds, recover 10 seconds, then repeat the cycle for a total of eight times in 4 minutes. I love to finish this 4-minute blast with a run. It really boosts my endurance and cardiovascular strength. Even on super busy days, I will warm up 10 minutes, do my 8 minutes of Tabata, and then cool down and stretch. It's a quick work-out that works!

# BUILDING MUSCLE/ADDING STRENGTH

## PUT THE KEY IN THE IGNITION:
## WHAT YOU NEED TO BUILD MUSCLE MASS

You've come so far. Now you want the strongest, hottest body you can have. And that's not about your scale weight; it's all about losing fat and building lean muscle. Here's how to pump up, along with some great recipes that will make that hard work worth working (out) for.

- Up and at 'Em

- HIIT It

- Take Some R&R

- Remember the 3:1 Ratio

- Go Low Carb—Low-Glycemic Carbs

- Eat More Foods, More Often

## UP AND AT 'EM

You can't build muscle if you don't work your muscles. They just don't build themselves. This might sound obvious, but sometimes folks confuse getting a cardiovascular workout (exercise for your heart and overall health) with what's needed for building muscle. While a run or walk (choose your own favorite cardio exercise) will do a world of good for your heart, none of the above will do much for gaining muscle mass. To get where you want to go, you must strength-train. That can mean using your own body weight, if you don't belong to a gym, or barbells and the like in your basement. Ladies, sorry, lifting 1- to 3-pound weights here isn't going to cut it. You need to challenge yourself more. Remember that old adage, no pain, no gain? Well, I'm going to revise it to, no strain, no muscle gain. I'm not saying go out and work to the point of pain, but you do have to be willing to get a little uncomfortable and put some real effort into it. But here's the gift: you should keep these intense bouts to 15- to 20-minute intervals. When eating a plant-based diet, for maximum benefit and less muscle wear-and-tear, keep the workouts intense but short. Unless you haven't exercised in years and years, you can handle a 5-, 8-, or even 10-pound hand weight. And you won't just build muscle with strength training, you'll also increase bone mass, decrease fat, increase cardiovascular fitness, and achieve a greater sense of overall wellbeing.

To develop muscle mass, try the method I've used. After I've increased the weight I use to where I can only do 12 reps, I will add on another plate, or go up 5 to 10 lbs when using dumbbells, and then I will do 10 reps. Once I can successfully do this, I will add a little more weight again, and perform 8 reps. After that, ideally, I add on additional weight and try my best to complete 6 reps. What I've found to be key is pushing myself to failure. It's all about using heavier weights, fewer reps, and slow, gentle movements. I make sure to slow down to really focus on my form while really squeezing the contraction to activate my muscles.

## HIIT IT

Generally, we want more muscle for power. And a great way to build power and get a little extra fat burn as well is through high-intensity interval training or HIIT. The basic idea is that you go really hard at an exercise in a 2 to 1 ratio of recovery time to work time. For example, walk or jog for 60 seconds after a 30-second sprint; do this for a total of 10 to 20 minutes—no longer. You could also try the Tabata Protocol I mentioned: do 20 seconds of high-intensity cardio, then 10 seconds rest, in a 4-minute cycle. You won't need more than 4 minutes of this every three days to be at peak. Always warm up first for a few minutes, stretch, and cool down properly to aid recovery.

Treadmills aren't a great choice for Tabata, but elliptical and rowing machines, stationary bikes, and the like all work well. Think about sprinters and how much muscle mass they have compared to long-distance runners, who are usually long and lean. That's what you'll get with this type of workout.

## TAKE SOME R&R

Did you know you don't build muscle at the gym? Well, it's true. You break down your muscles there and stimulate them as well, but they grow during your recovery time. So sleep is important here, as is making sure that you don't overtrain. So to revise the old adage again, if you want to gain, don't overtrain. Though there are times when you can overtrain on purpose (in advance of a long vacation where you won't be exercising and you will be getting plenty of rest), it's generally something you wish to avoid if your goal is to build, not continue to destroy, muscle tissue.

A few tips that will help. Aim for 3-minute rests between sets. Exercise individual muscle groups once a week. When training hard and continually, take a week off from exercise every few months.

## REMEMBER THE 3:1 RATIO

Just as you can't build muscle without the proper exercise, it's pretty hard to add muscle without adequate protein supplies. Eating in a ratio of 3 to 1, protein to carbs, is what successful bodybuilders frequently aim to do. Eating some protein immediately after a workout (within 15 minutes) will decrease muscle soreness; eating protein immediately before and after exercise is believed to be beneficial to increasing muscle mass and sustaining immune function during intense training periods. Marrying a protein with a high-quality carbohydrate gives you even more bang for your buck, increasing muscle protein synthesis, replacing glycogen stores more quickly, and aiding in recovery time.

***Top Your Tank:*** *Brown rice protein powder, hemp, nuts, seeds, buckwheat, sea vegetables, quinoa, spirulina, cholorella, wheatgrass, and chickpeas (cooked).*

⭐ **Power It Up!**

Hemp is a highly sustainable plant that can be used for many different purposes. High in vitamin E, it is a powerful antioxidant that helps further speed recovery. It also contains anti-inflammatory properties that help with soft tissue repair. Hemp seeds contain all the essential amino acids, are highly digestible, and are one of the highest sources of complete protein of all plant-based foods. Hemp is also a great source of dietary fiber, magnesium, iron, zinc, and potassium.

## GO LOW CARB—LOW-GLYCEMIC CARBS

Remember the low carb craze of the eighties? Well it turns out, some carbs—like a lot of the ones on this plan—are good for you. They key is to choose carbs that are lower on the glycemic index (GI). Sound like more mumbo jumbo? It's not. The GI is simply a measure of the effects of carbohydrates on blood sugar levels. Refined white carbs are those that give us the least amount of energy; carbohydrates that have a lower glycemic index give us sustained energy and steady blood sugar levels. If insulin levels are in check you'll find it easier to burn fat, and less fat will sit around in storage, obscuring those beautiful muscles you're building up. Go nuts for nuts (unless you're allergic); they're a low GI food that will give you healthy fat, antioxidants, protein, and extra calories. As such, they are a great source of energy for intense training and a good source of nutrients beneficial to athletes. Plus, cashews are said to be a natural antidepressant because they contain niacin and tryptophan. Half a cup provides about 470 mg tryptophan.

*Top Your Tank:* *Asparagus, artichoke, cabbage, oatmeal, okra, nuts, turnip greens, watercress, and zucchini.*

## EAT MORE FOODS, MORE OFTEN

For the best benefit, try to eat small meals, every two to three hours. Calorie deficits during training can actually derail both your progress and the health benefits of this type of exercise. So don't be afraid to eat up! Make sure to vary your food sources so as to avoid any nutrient deficiencies; focus on iron and calcium-rich foods like broccoli and spinach. And don't forget to drink up. Hydration is key to muscle recovery. Drink small sips throughout your workout, every 10 to 15 minutes or so, and make sure to fill up on water right after. Eat a piece of fruit and protein source while refilling your water tank, and you'll be taking the best care of those worked muscles.

I love snacking on dulse, a sea vegetable, while sipping water post workout. Sea veggies taste salty not from sodium, but from potassium, so it's perfect for replenishing electrolytes. And if you have access to Thai young baby coconuts, fresh, rather than from a can or box, that's living water packed with natural electrolytes. So good, and good for you!

*Top Your Tank:* Buckwheat, brown rice protein powder, dark leafy greens, hemp protein, flaxseed, pumpkin and sunflower seeds, sea vegetables, walnuts, and peanut butter (cooked).

## EATING FOR MUSCLE-BUILDING: THE RECIPES

These recipes are designed to build muscle mass using plant based protein sources. The bars and cookies make for great snacks that you can carry with you easily. And the shakes pair well with lean animal proteins like bison and wild-caught, low-mercury fish.

### Basic Protein Shake

**PHASES 2 AND 3 BREAKFAST OR SNACK**
MAKES 1 PINT, 1 SERVING

This is a basic protein shake recipe made with either hemp protein or buckwheat groats that have been soaked in at least double the amount of filtered water for 8 hours or so. You can also use Buckwheat Crispies (which are groats that have been soaked and then dried in a dehydrator; for the recipe, check out page 66 of *Ani's Raw Food Kitchen*).

> 2 tablespoons hemp protein powder or buckwheat groats, soaked, or in the form of Buckwheat Crispies
>
> ½ cup greens, any type
>
> 1 cup banana, about 1 whole
>
> 1½ cup coconut water or filtered water, to desired consistency
>
> ½ cup ice

Place all ingredients into high-speed blender. Blend until smooth.

Best enjoyed immediately, but it will keep in fridge for one day stored in sealed container, ideally glass.

## Green Blueberry Coconut Shake

**PHASES 2 AND 3 BREAKFAST OR SNACK**
MAKES 1 PINT, 1 SERVING

A variation of the **Basic Protein Shake**. Berries and vanilla are added to create a new and delicious flavor.

**1 batch Basic Protein Shake**

**½ cup blueberries**

**1 tablespoon alcohol-free vanilla extract, or seeds from one whole vanilla bean**

Place all ingredients into high-speed blender. Blend until smooth.

Best enjoyed immediately, but it will keep in fridge, if tightly sealed, for one day.

## Robert's Vegan Bodybuilding Trail Mix

COURTESY OF ROBERT CHEEKE

**PHASE 3 BREAKFAST OR SNACK**
MAKES 4 SERVINGS

This is a recipe from Robert's book *Vegan Bodybuilding & Fitness* that is delicious. It's packed with nuts, seeds, and dried fruit. It's also tasty as a morning granola cereal served in a bowl with the nonanimal milk of your choice.

**½ cup almonds**

**½ cup walnuts**

**½ cup pecans**

**½ cup cashews**

**¼ cup pumpkin seeds**

**¼ cup sesame seeds**

**¼ cup hemp seeds**

**¼ cup sunflower seeds**

**½ cup dates**

**½ cup raisins**

Mix into a bowl, serve, and enjoy!

# Robert's Vegan Weight Gainer

COURTESY OF ROBERT CHEEKE

**MAINTENANCE PHASE**
MAKES 1 SERVING

Here's another great recipe from *Vegan Bodybuilding & Fitness* that focuses on building muscle mass. L-glutamine plays a major role in DNA synthesis and transports nitrogen into muscle tissue to replenish nitrogen loss from excessive muscle training; it also helps speed recovery.

- **2 cups hemp milk**
- **3 tablespoons organic peanut butter or organic almond butter**
- **1 whole organic avocado**
- **½ cup oats**
- **1 tablespoon pea protein powder**
- **1 tablespoon hemp protein powder**
- **1 tablespoon rice protein powder**
- **2 tablespoons flax oil**
- **½ organic chocolate bar**
- **Add ice and water as needed**

Blend, serve, and enjoy!

# Robert's Post-Workout Power Pudding

COURTESY OF ROBERT CHEEKE

**PHASE 3 BREAKFAST OR SNACK**
MAKES 2 SERVINGS

- **1 cup almond milk**
- **1 cup dates**
- **2 tablespoons pea protein powder**
- **1 tablespoon rice protein powder**
- **¼ cup hemp seeds**

¼ cup chia seeds

pinch of cinnamon

Add water or more almond milk as needed for consistency.

Blend, serve, and enjoy!

## Chocolate Protein Pudding

PHASES **2** AND **3** BREAKFAST OR SNACK
MAKES 1 SERVING

A delicious chocolate pudding kids love that's secretly filled with spinach and spirulina. Its creamy richness comes from blended banana and the natural heart-healthy fat of avocado.

½ cup avocado, from about ½ whole

½ cup banana, from about ½ whole

¼ cup spinach, rinsed well

1 tablespoon hemp protein powder

1 tablespoon cacao powder

1 teaspoon spirulina powder

1 cup Thai baby coconut water, or filtered water, to desired consistency

Place all ingredients into your high-speed blender. Blend until smooth.

Enjoy immediately.

Will keep for one day in fridge sealed in airtight container, ideally glass.

## Basic Protein Oatmeal

MAINTENANCE PHASE
MAKES 2 SERVINGS

Oatmeal is rich in complex, energy-sustaining, carbohydrates. It is low in fat and high in fiber, plus it is economically priced. Hemp protein has a strong flavor, so you may want to add it to your oatmeal gradually to suit your own tastes and liking. This is a basic recipe for my easy-to-make raw oatmeal.

Add your favorite flavors or ingredients to make endless variations from this starting point.

**1 cup raw oat groats, soaked overnight and rinsed well**

**1 cup buckwheat groats, soaked overnight and rinsed well**

**¼ cup pitted dates, or 1 cup banana, from about 1 whole**

**2 tablespoons hemp protein powder, or brown rice protein powder**

Place all ingredients into your food processor. Process into a creamy texture that's like cooked oatmeal.

**Try these variations:**

**Apple Cinnamon**—Add ½ cup chopped apple and sprinkle with cinnamon powder.

**French Vanilla**—Add 1 tablespoon alcohol-free vanilla extract, or the seeds from 1 whole fresh vanilla bean.

**Chocolate Crunch**—Add 1 tablespoon cacao powder and 1 tablespoon cacao nibs.

**Cinnamon Raisin**—Add 2 tablespoons raisins with a dash of cinnamon powder.

**Butter Pecan**—Add 1 tablespoon coconut oil and 1 tablespoon pecan pieces.

**Fruit and Kream**—Serve topped with strawberries, blueberries, banana, and your favorite mylk made by blending a handful of raw nuts with 4 to 6 cups of filtered water. Or, add coconut, almond, or rice milk found at most grocery stores.

**Maple Walnut**—Top with 1 to 2 tablespoons crushed walnuts and 1 tablespoon maple syrup, to taste.

 ## Power Cookies

**PHASE 3 SNACK**
MAKES 4 SERVINGS OR
ABOUT ONE DOZEN 1-TABLESPOON-SIZED COOKIES

Buckwheat is the source for low-fat protein in these cookies, and it adds a light and crunchy texture. To create different textures and tastes, swap out the buckwheat with the same amount of cashews or almonds. Cacao and dates provide lasting energy, while mesquite, hemp, and brown rice protein powder add more protein.

> 1 cup pitted semisoft dates, packed, like medjool
>
> 1 tablespoon almond butter, raw
>
> 3 tablespoons hemp protein powder, or brown rice protein powder
>
> 2 tablespoons mesquite powder, or cacao or cocoa powder
>
> 1 tablespoon cacao nibs
>
> ½ cup Buckwheat Crispies (groats that have been soaked and then dried in a dehydrator; for the recipe, check out page 66 of *Ani's Raw Food Kitchen*)

Place dates and almond butter into food processor and pulse to mix well until the dates break down into small pieces. Next, add hemp and either mesquite or cocoa powder. Process to mix well. Last, add cacao nibs and Buckwheat Crispies, and pulse gently to mix. Scoop dough into 1-tablespoon sized balls and flatten into cookies.

Will keep for weeks in the fridge stored in airtight container. Makes for great travel food at room temperature, too.

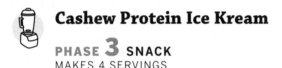

## Cashew Protein Ice Kream

**PHASE 3 SNACK**
MAKES 4 SERVINGS

A creamy, dreamy, frozen treat made by blending together frozen fruit and soaked cashews. For a sweeter taste, add your favorite sweetener. Cashews, and generally all nuts, are high in tryptophan, and a couple handfuls of cashew nuts is said to naturally treat depression. So eat up and feel happy!

> 1 cup cashews, soaked overnight, rinsed well
>
> 3 cups frozen banana, pineapple, or your favorite fruit
>
> 2 to 3 tablespoons agave nectar, maple syrup, date syrup, or stevia, to taste, optional

Place all ingredients into your high-speed blender. Use tamper to push food into the blades to blend smooth. Enjoy immediately, or to firm up, scoop into container, seal, and place in freezer overnight.

## Basic Protein Bars

PHASE **3** SNACK
MAKES 4 BARS, 4 SERVINGS

These bars travel well, and I love carrying them to the gym to enjoy post workout. This recipe is also the base for two other great options made by adding in a few extra ingredients.

**1 cup almonds, or your favorite nuts, dry**

**3 tablespoons hemp protein powder, or brown rice protein powder**

**1 tablespoon maca powder**

**1 cup pitted semisoft dates, like medjool**

**pinch of sea salt, to taste, optional**

Place almonds into a food processor; process into small pieces. Add hemp protein powder and maca, and pulse lightly to mix. Add dates and process to mix into a batter.

Dust a baking tray with about ¼ cup almond meal, or line with plastic wrap. Press batter into the tray to form large square or rectangle of desired thickness. Flip dough out of the tray onto a cutting board. Cut into bar shapes.

These bars will keep for weeks at room temperature and will keep for at least a month when refrigerated in a sealed container.

## Chocolate Crunch Protein Bars

PHASE **3** SNACK
MAKES 4 BARS

**1 batch Basic Protein Bars, above**

**1 tablespoon cacao powder**

**2 tablespoons cacao nibs**

**pinch sea salt, optional**

Place almonds into a food processor; process into small pieces. Add hemp protein powder, maca, and cacao powder, and pulse lightly to mix. Add dates and process to mix into a batter. Add nibs last, and pulse gently to mix.

Dust a baking tray with a couple tablespoons of cacao powder. Press batter into tray to desired thickness. Flip dough out of the tray onto a cutting board. Cut into four bars.

Bars will keep for weeks at room temperature and will keep at least a month when refrigerated in a sealed container.

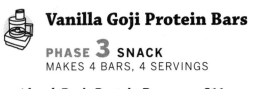

## Vanilla Goji Protein Bars

PHASE **3** SNACK
MAKES 4 BARS, 4 SERVINGS

1 batch **Basic Protein Bars**, page 211

1 tablespoon vanilla extract, or the seeds from 1 fresh vanilla bean

¼ cup goji berries

pinch sea salt, to taste, optional

Place almonds into food processor, and process into small pieces. Add hemp protein powder, maca, and vanilla, and pulse lightly to mix. Add dates and process to mix into a batter. Add goji berries last, and pulse gently to mix.

Dust a baking tray with 2 or 3 tablespoons of almond meal, or line with plastic wrap. Press batter into tray. Flip dough out of the tray onto a cutting board. Cut into four bars.

Bars will keep for weeks at room temperature and will keep at least a month when refrigerated in sealed container.

**START YOUR ENGINES:** THE MUSCLE BUILDING WORKOUT

If you can't get to a gym, simple exercises like push-ups, chin-ups, crunches, squats, and lunges work great for building muscle mass. I like to do them controlled and slow, while really focusing on squeezing the contraction to engage the muscle fully. Plus, I do two or three sets to failure. Remember muscles build while you rest, so when working out to build muscle mass, give yourself a full 48 hours to recover. Work hard. Don't just go through the motions here. You'll gain nothing and cheat yourself at the same time.

# INCREASING FLEXIBILITY

## PUT THE KEY IN THE IGNITION:
### WAYS TO INCREASE FLEXIBILITY

Life is all about balance, isn't it? And building strength and endurance should go hand-in-hand with making sure all your parts are in good, supple working order. Here're a few ways keep your joints and tissues "well-oiled" and in good working condition.

- Avoid Inflammatory Foods; Embrace Plants
- Women, Check Your Hormones
- Just A Spoonful of . . . Vinegar
- Get the Connection: MSM and Sulfur
- Keep Circulating
- It's a Stretch

## AVOID INFLAMMATORY FOODS; EMBRACE PLANTS

If you want to be your own personal flexible best, you shouldn't ingest foods known to cause inflammation in the body. Inflammation is how your body reacts to injury, whether it's from exercise or another source—like your diet. Inflammation prevents cell regeneration and gradually tears down tissues. It is caused by an increase in free radicals, poor diet, food allergies and sensitivities, sustained stress, and hormonal shifts. It can nestle in the muscles and the joints, leading to stiffness, which will make you want to move even less. This creates a vicious cycle; you want no part of it. To turn down the heat, you need to avoid the following foods:

- Highly refined carbohydrates and sugar, white flour, modified fats, and artificial colorings
- Animal proteins
- Common allergy foods, like soy, corn, wheat, and dairy*

* Dairy products are believed to be one of the most notorious offenders in creating joint inflammation.

What should you eat? By now you know the answer I'm going to give you: plants. Norwegian researchers put 27 people with rheumatoid arthritis on a vegetarian diet for a year. After that time, the participants reported less joint pain, swelling, and stiffness than those who ate a traditional omnivore diet. Here are a few more to enjoy frequently.

**Top Your Tank:** *Chlorella, dark, leafy greens, nuts, sea vegetables, raw cacao, and spirulina.*

## ☆ POWER IT UP: *Chlorella*

Chlorella, a freshwater algae from Japan, is one of my favorite foods you are likely to never have heard of before now. It has more chlorophyll than any other plant or animal, a great amount of B12, and consists of almost 70 percent protein (more than animal products and more digestible). It has 19 amino acids and over 20 vitamins and minerals. Chlorella has some other pretty great benefits, too, because it: relieves inflammation, supports healthy weight loss, and improves digestion and elimination.

Chlorella comes in a powdered form, and the powder is also pressed into tablets. I love munching on the tablets as snacks throughout the day and post-workout because I love the flavor, texture, and know how good it is for me.

## WOMEN, CHECK YOUR HORMONES

Perimenopausal women often experience joint pain. Declining estrogen levels during this lifestage are believed to be the culprit, as estrogen has anti-inflammatory effects within the body. So falling levels can exacerbate symptoms. Have your physician check this out, but many will repeat what I say here: the key dietary recommendation to relieve symptoms is to increase plant foods, especially those high in phyto (plant) estrogens and natural progesterone. If your doctor agrees that you should be adding these to your daily diet, then enjoy filling your tank with the foods listed below.

***Top Your Tank:*** *Alfalfa grass, apple, barley grass, berries, carrots, celery, cherries, fennel, flaxseed, garbanzos (cooked or sprouts), green beans, oats, olives, parsley, plums, red clover, saffron, soy (cooked), seeds (pumpkin, sunflower, sesame, and poppy), and sprouted rye.*

## JUST A SPOONFUL OF . . . VINEGAR

Even though I love Mary Poppins, she should have been singing the praises of vinegar, not sugar. I imagine most kids and even grown-ups might pucker up at this thought, but if you read the Power Packed on page 6, you already know this is a food well-worth playing "dress-up" with each day. For years, natural health followers have sworn by apple cider vinegar as a treatment for arthritis. Although there is no scientific research that supports the use of vinegar for increasing flexibility, there is considerable anecdotal (read: real people swearing by it) information out there saying it doesn't hurt to give it a try. I remember a science class experiment in elementary school where we placed a turkey bone into vinegar for a while, and when we took it out, it was flexible! I grew up a gymnast, and, even back then, I realized vinegar would help my flexibility and performance.

## GET THE CONNECTION: MSM AND SULFUR

MSM (big-word alert: methylsulfonylmethane) is a powerful anti-inflammatory and antioxidant; it is also a great source of sulfur (34 percent sulfur content by weight). Sulfur bonds are essential structural features in all connective tissue, and it is believed that sulfur compounds—like MSM, glucosamine, and chondroitin—have protective benefits in protecting against joint and cartilage deterioration. When amino acids, in particular vitamin C, are present, the body metabolizes MSM to sulfur. MSM is also believed to aid with circulation, increasing blood flow throughout your body.

***Top Your Tank:*** *Asparagus, brussels sprouts, garlic, onions, kale, wheat germ, and legumes (cooked).*

## KEEP CIRCULATING

Bridgette Mars, author of 12 books and a nutritional consultant, names seven spices and herbs that increase circulation while making us feel warmer (they're great to enjoy in the cold winter months). They and their benefits include the following: black pepper (antiseptic and antioxidant), cardamom (expectorant, opens the respiratory passages), cayenne (high in vitamin C, relieves chills, coughs, congestion), cinnamon (antiseptic, digestive tonic), garlic (vasodilator, improves circulation), ginger (antioxidant, antiseptic), and horseradish (high in vitamin C, aids digestion of fatty foods, a strong decongestant). So, in addition to decreasing or eliminating inflammatory foods, increasing these seven spices and herbs will keep your blood circulating, bringing fresh blood and oxygen to all parts of your body to help heal and repair, build, and increase overall flexibility.

## IT'S A DAILY STRETCH

I've given you some tips on what to eat and what nutrients are important for joint and muscle flexibility. But just like you can't build muscle without exercise, you can't enjoy the benefits of these various tips if you don't actually stretch your muscles. The best way, I think, is to do yoga. Any kind will do, to my mind. You just have to do it, and do it every day. Stretching isn't just good for your joints and improving flexibility, it also helps you to relax, improves posture, relieves pain and stiffness, enhances energy, and increases circulation. We can all benefit from stretching, even if it's as simple as a stretch getting up from our desk at work each hour for five minutes. Stretching is yet another one of those amazing multitaskers I like so much.

## EATING FOR FLEXIBILITY: THE RECIPES

These juice recipes will fill your body with tons of beneficial nutrients, while helping to increase circulation and flexibility by getting more oxygen-filled blood into all parts of your body. You will need a juicer to make these juice recipes, but if you don't have a juicer, your blender will work, too. Just put ingredients into the blender with as much filtered water as desired. You can choose to strain out the fiber with a sieve or filtration bag or cheese cloth, or just drink up!

## Angela's Chocolate Milk Juice

COURTESY OF ANGELA STOKES-MONARCH

**PHASES 1, 2, AND 3**
VEGETABLE JUICES CAN BE ADDED TO ANY DAY,
ANY PHASE.
MAKES 1 SERVING

Angela says this juice tastes "just" like chocolate milk (depending on your taste-buds), and it can be made sweeter with more carrots or even with apples if desired.

**1 bunch spinach**

**1 head romaine lettuce**

**6 medium carrots**

**2 apples, as desired, optional**

Juice 'em up and serve.

## Angela's Pine Green Juice

COURTESY OF ANGELA STOKES-MONARCH

**PHASES 1, 2, AND 3**
VEGETABLE JUICES CAN BE ADDED TO ANY DAY,
ANY PHASE.
MAKES 1 SERVING

Angela says this is one of her favorite juice combinations—greens with pineapple. You can really use any greens you have available, then add in the pineapple juice at the last moment before drinking because the enzymes in the pineapple start to break down the green juice very quickly. This same recipe also makes a great shake, if you want to blend rather than juice. When blending, use only a quarter of the ingredients with filtered water, as needed, to desired consistency.

**½ bunch celery**

**1 cucumber**

**½ bunch parsley**

**1 big bunch of whichever leafy greens you have available: lettuces, spinach, kale**

**½ to 1 pineapple, to taste**

Juice and enjoy. Best enjoyed immediately.

## Tonya's Ultimate Combo Smoothie

COURTESY OF TONYA ZAVASTA

**PHASES 2 AND 3 BREAKFAST**
MAKES 1 SERVING

Ultimate combos are not restricted to the fast food drive-thru. Here is one of my favorite summer recipes, incorporating the first melons and figs of summer.

**1½ cups peeled, chunked watermelon**

**1 cup fresh ripe figs**

**2 medium to large leaves of Lacinato kale or Swiss chard, stems removed**

Thoroughly blend all ingredients in a Vita-Mix or other blender and pour into medium-sized glasses. Grab a straw and enjoy.

## Penni's Simple Mango Gazpacho

COURTESY OF PENNI SHELTON

**PHASES 2 AND 3**
4 SERVINGS

This sweet and savory soup is so creamy and delicious, you'll almost forget you're eating something healthy!

**2 cups fresh mangoes, diced**

**2 cups freshly squeezed orange juice**

**1 cup cucumber, peeled, seeded, and chopped**

**1 small red bell pepper, seeded and chopped**

**2 garlic cloves, minced**

**1 small jalapeño pepper, seeded and minced, optional**

3 tablespoons fresh lime juice

2 tablespoons fresh cilantro, chopped (basil or mint would also be nice)

1 to 2 tablespoons cold pressed, organic extra virgin olive oil

1 teaspoon onion powder

Himalayan sea salt and freshly ground black pepper, to taste

red onion, chopped, for garnish

avocado, sliced, for garnish

Reserve a bit of the mango, cucumber, red pepper, and cilantro to use as the final garnish, if desired. Process the remaining ingredients in a high-speed blender until smooth and creamy. Taste and adjust with salt and pepper to taste. Refrigerate until ready to serve.

Pour into bowls and garnish for soup. This can easily be poured into a glass and enjoyed as a savory, sweet smoothie.

## Tonya's Russian Borscht
COURTESY OF TONYA ZAVASTA

PHASE **3** LUNCH, DINNER, OR SNACK
MAKES 1 SERVING

Tonya shares her favorite borscht recipe, filled with vegetable juices and refreshing cucumber, beets, and creamy avocado.

Juice enough of the following vegetables to equal:

¾ cups tomato juice

½ cup carrot juice

¼ cup cucumber juice

¼ cup celery juice

¼ cup lemon juice

You needn't worry about exact measurements—just shoot enough of each vegetable through the juicer to equal the approximate amount. Pour the juices into a bowl, adding:

½ cup shredded beet

½ cup minced red pepper

½ medium cucumber, chopped

1½ scallions, minced

½ large avocado, cubed

1 tomato, diced

2 tablespoons parsley, chopped

dash of cumin, salt, and cayenne pepper, to taste

Stir together and ENJOY!

 ## Philip's Tangy Avocado and Jicama Salsa

COURTESY OF PHILIP MCCLUSKEY

PHASE **3** LUNCH, DINNER, OR SNACK
MAKES 1 SERVING

Creamy, crunchy, salty, sweet: this salad is almost a salsa, and it's definitely perfection. With supermarkets carrying avocados and jicama all year round nowadays, it's a pleasure you can savor in any season, but it's particularly refreshing during the summer months. Plus, it really couldn't be any easier to make!

1 cup jicama, peeled and diced

1 cup avocado, pitted and halved, scored into small pieces and scooped out of their skins into the bowl, from about 1 whole

¼ cup red onion, finely chopped

¼ teaspoon minced garlic, optional

⅛ to ¼ teaspoon (or more to taste) chili powder

1 tablespoon lime juice

1 teaspoon lemon juice

1 teaspoon fresh or dried cilantro

generous pinch sea salt (or to taste)

Mix all ingredients together in a bowl. Keep covered in the fridge until ready to serve.

# Green Papaya Salad

**PHASES 2 AND 3** **MEAL OR SNACK**
MAKES 4 SERVINGS

This recipe first appeared in *Ani's Raw Food Essentials*, page 157. While any of my cookbooks provide recipes that can help you incorporate more life-giving whole foods into your diet, this particular recipe is one of my favorites.

## DRESSING

2 tablespoons lime juice, from about 1 whole

2 tablespoons agave, or your favorite syrup

## SALAD

4 cups papayas, julienned

2 cups carrots, shredded

2 red chilies, sliced thinly, to taste

## GARNISH

½ cup fresh cilantro, chopped

½ cup fresh basil, chopped

⅓ cup almonds, chopped

Whisk together the lime juice and agave in large mixing bowl.

Add salad ingredients; toss to mix well. Set aside to marinate for 15 to 20 minutes.

To serve, top with herbs and almonds.

Will keep for two days in fridge.

# Penni's Pasta with Tomatoes, Arugula, Capers, and Olives

COURTESY OF PENNI SHELTON

**PHASE 3** LUNCH, DINNER, OR SNACK
MAKES 1 SERVING

6 plum or Roma tomatoes, seeded and chopped

⅓ cup Kalamata olives, halved, pitted

⅓ cup arugula, chopped, packed

2 tablespoons capers, drained

1 tablespoon organic, cold pressed extra virgin olive oil

2 cloves garlic, minced

½ teaspoon crushed red pepper

Himalayan sea salt and fresh black pepper, to taste

fresh basil leaves

2 zucchini squash (or carrots, parsnip, turnip, etc.)

Toss the first seven ingredients in a medium bowl; season to taste with salt and pepper. Let stand for at least 30 minutes for the flavors to develop.

Use a spiral slicer, or julienne, to create zucchini noodles. Gently toss the tomato mixture into the noodles and serve with a garnish of fresh basil leaves.

## START YOUR ENGINES: THE FLEXIBILITY WORKOUT

Don't forget to hydrate any time you stretch or work out. And just because you're stretching with yoga doesn't mean you're not working your body. It still needs fluids to keep you as fluid as possible. Do some sort of stretching routine daily, and you'll be limber and loose in no time.

I like to sweat daily, and prior to running, biking, or hiking, I'll stretch for 5 to 10 minutes. But after my workouts, I love stretching for anywhere from 10 to 30 minutes. This is when I'll do my yoga and sun salutations, when my body is warmed up and limber. Plus, the stretching helps with muscle recovery post workout.

## ☆ Immune-Proofing the Body

As you've likely noticed, enjoying fresh, natural, and whole plant-based foods boosts our immune system because we are fueling up on super-duper dense nutrients, antioxidants, vitamins, minerals, amino acids, enzymes, and all good-for-us ingredients that help us fight off poor health. Any and all of the recipes in this book are great for boosting our immune system before getting on an airplane or entering other contained areas when we may be surrounded by less healthy people.

I travel frequently for work, which means sleeping in hotels and jetting about. Usually, I don't rest as well when I'm on the road; my exercise routine is thrown off; and it may be challenging to eat as well as I do when I'm at home. So, before and during travel, I like to blast myself full of high levels of antioxidants, vitamins, and minerals to help keep me at my best. I usually avoid alcohol if possible, especially on the plane. Rather, I'll try to drink a liter of water for every hour on a plane. That keeps me hydrated and moving because I often have to get up to go to the restroom. Plus, that open area near the restroom is a great place to stretch.

I've listed some things I like to pack in my suitcase in Chapter 7, and I've learned to only carry on, even when going overseas for six weeks. I'll carry nori (fits flat in outside pocket of my suitcase), chlorella tablets, dried sea vegetables (they hydrate to three to four times their size), hemp protein powder, green powders like dehydrated barley grass or wheat grass, dried fruits like goji berries and golden berries, dehydrated flax crackers, and snacks that can remain unrefrigerated for a while like carrots, jicama, cucumbers, lemon, and avocado.

And, for several days before travel, and during travel, I pump myself full of green vegetable juices to immune-proof myself.

Here are foods and nutrients I especially like to enjoy prior to, during, and post travel to keep me as healthy and vibrant as possible.

**Top Your Tank:** *High-antioxidant foods like fruits, veggies, nuts, and seeds that are particularly high in vitamins A, C, and E. MUFAs from avocado and nuts. Goji berries, camu camu, acai, spirulina, turmeric, and high-quality proteins (their amino acids glutamine and arginine may stimulate the immune system).*

# THE UNPROCESSED LIFE

**You've cleaned up your diet.** Bravo! Now, perhaps I can inspire you to also clean up the rest of your life so that you're living exactly the life you deserve: healthy, joyous, and fun. The very first thing I'll say here before diving into tips on living an unprocessed life is this: live your life!

I've heard it said that often we put on excess weight because we may be waiting to live the life we want. So, now that you've blasted away those boundaries and feel energized and look amazing, commit to trying something new you've always wanted to do. Start by taking a martial arts class; learn ballet; get out hiking or rollerblading; try painting, singing, or even sky diving! We create our own biggest barriers, and it's our thoughts that cause doubt and fear. Let that all go, and live your life to the fullest!

## LIVE AN UNPROCESSED LIFE

Now that you've dissolved away crusted-on engine crud, detoxed, cleaned, and greened yourself from the inside out, we want to make sure you don't bring contaminants and junk that will bog you down back into the mix.

Poisonous chemicals can enter our bodies through the air we breathe, be absorbed from the fabrics that sit on our skin, and even taken in from the water we shower with each day. I fight back by applying the same principles I use when choosing unprocessed foods when picking products to put on my skin, in my hair, and into my home and work environments. Choose whole, recognizable, nontoxic ingredients that have not been manufactured in a factory. It's that simple.

## THE UGLY TRUTH ABOUT BEAUTY

Toxic poisons are found in most personal care products like lotions and makeup. Once we realize this, we can then choose to read labels, to become familiar with ingredients, and then avoid putting things on our skin that would be poisonous to eat. After all, our skin is our largest organ. Whatever we put on our skin is absorbed into our body. I use edible oils from my kitchen as moisturizers, like hemp, flax, and coconut (that's my favorite). I rub coconut oil through the ends of my hair to defrizz it, and it leaves a delicious scent. As you know, avocado is a heart-healthy fat. But if you have an avocado that's too ripe to eat, mash it up and make a mask to spread over your face, or rub it through your hair. The healthy fat within it will add incredible moisture to your face and hair. Papaya, pineapple, or grapefruit have great fruit enzymes for exfoliating the skin. My earlier books have a lot of toxin-free natural recipes for your skin; two of my favorites are Banana Wrap for Moist Silky Skin and Fruit Salad to Feed Your Skin from *Ani's Raw Food Desserts*.

### Banana Wrap for Moist Silky Skin

Biotin is the most important B vitamin for our skin. It forms the basis of skin, nail, and hair cells and gives skin a healthy glow while hydrating cells and increasing overall skin tone. Bananas are a great source of both biotin and potassium, which helps us maintain healthy, beautiful skin and hair, is great for wrinkles, and plumps up our skin.

**1 very ripe banana**

**2 tablespoons olive oil**

Mash the banana with a fork in a small bowl. Add the oil and mix well.

Fill a mixing bowl with very warm filtered water. Place a face towel in the water.

Spread the banana mixture on your face and neck. Cover with paper or tissue, and top with the warm damp towel.

Relax on the bed, couch, or better yet, in the tub, for 20 to 30 minutes.

Shower with warm water to remove.

## 🄰 Feed Your Skin a Fruit Salad

Pineapple is delicious in many raw desserts. But did you know that it's super beneficial for your skin, too? Pineapple has anti-inflammatory properties, is a mild astringent, and its enzymes dissolve skin's dead cells and dirt. It's a great component of this fruit salad skin mask, which also includes bananas to make our skin smooth and soft; kiwi, which is high in vitamin C and enzymes; and honeydew melon to cool and hydrate. If you have fruit that's too ripe to eat, try making this salad for your skin. Apply the mask pool- or ocean-side— it's sticky and fun.

**2 cups pineapple, peeled and chopped**

**2 cups honeydew melon, chopped**

**1 banana, chopped**

**2 kiwi fruit, peeled and chopped**

Combine all the ingredients in the food processor and process into a lumpy texture. Apply to body and face and leave on for 20 to 30 minutes.

Rinse in an outdoor shower, with a hose, or in the ocean and enjoy smooth radiant skin!

## MAKE YOUR OWN CLEANING PRODUCTS

Ever notice when walking through a grocery store how you can smell the aisle with all the cleaning products? Well, that's because the chemicals are outgassing through the containers they are stored in. Keep these in your home and you'll be inhaling the same toxic fumes daily.

Cleansers are easy to make. And doing so saves money and keeps you from bringing more poison into your environment. It's as simple as using the same ingredients we used to dissolve crud from the inside of your body: lemons, vinegar, and coconut oil. And baking soda works as a great scrub for stainless steel and cast iron. You'll find more nontoxic cleaning recipes in *Ani's Raw Food Desserts* and *Ani's Raw Food Asia*, as well as a list of poisonous ingredients commonly found in cleaning products. If you want even more, additional nontoxic cleanser recipes can be found in *Ani's Raw Food Essentials*.

## BREATHE CLEAN AIR

The Environmental Protection Agency (EPA) warns us that indoor air quality is our number one environmental health problem. As I stated earlier, the EPA estimates indoor air can be 2 to 10 times more hazardous than outdoor air, even in polluted cities. This is due to the chemicals we store under our bathroom sink, the outgassing of fabrics on our furniture, and volatile organic compounds (VOCs) found in the paint on our walls.

I'm of Korean decent and have been trained from day 1 to leave my shoes at the door to avoid tracking in residual pesticides and crud from outside. HEPA-filter vacuums filter out dust, bacteria, pollen, and Kanga's dog dander, and my shower curtains are PVC-free to avoid toxins that can disrupt my hormones. A NASA study found plants remove 96 percent of harmful carbon monoxide from a closed room. So it's no surprise that I've got a ton of green plants in my home that help clean and filter my indoor air (I was striving to recreate a Bali rainforest here in my Los Angeles home).

## LIVE SIMPLY

Now that you've started to unprocess your diet, beauty products, cleansers, and even the air you breathe, next up is to let go of anything that may be weighing you down, energetically. Living the unprocessed life means letting go of excess weight in the rest of your life: in your house, closet, office, basement, garage, car—you get the picture. In Asian culture, we practice feng shui, an ancient Chinese system of improving life by placing items in a specific way (and also leaving open space) to allow the flow of energy. Letting go of things we don't use, don't need, or haven't used in the past six months means opening up physical and energetic space to allow new energy to enter and flow freely. Enjoy living more simply.

I went through a period several years ago when I sold my four-story Victorian and let go of all the furnishings in my five-bedroom house. It was amazing to realize how much energy and history I had been lugging around with me. Letting it all go made me feel lighter, freer, fresher, open, and ready to take on new experiences and adventures. This may sound extreme, but for the next year, everything I owned fit into a carry-on suitcase. I'd have to let go of something old to make room for something new. I realized how having lots of possessions had taken up a lot of my brain space because I would have to think about them, take care of them, keep track of them, and keep them safe. After letting it all go, suddenly, I had brain space and power to think, do, and attract whatever I wanted. It was life-changing and completely liberating.

## REDUCE, REUSE, RECYCLE

Not only is this philosophy good for our planet, it saves a ton of money, which means fewer bills to pay and less stress overall. The less stuff we clutter ourselves with, the less we have to sell our time away to pay for everything we've purchased, leaving us with more time to spend with family and friends. Live for your life, not for a paycheck. When living life simply and cleanly, you're avoiding the processed life and being weighed down with extra stuff none of us really needs.

## AVOID TV

I already told you I think this is one key to happiness. Nontoxic living is just as much about avoiding toxic thoughts, which is hard to do when one is glued to the TV screen. Avoiding the processed life is avoiding a life that's been prewritten for you—avoiding a life filled with junk mail, junk TV, junk thoughts. All this bombardment wears you down both physically and mentally.

I haven't had a TV for about 20 years now. And a growing concern is that our youth are constantly plugged into watching TV, texting, playing video games, listening to iPods; they're constantly bombarded with information. The bad news is that this overstimulation leaves little time for their brains to be creative. Instead, the TV tells them (and us) what to think, which is why I call it a tell-a-vision. The vision we all develop, though, may not be our own; instead we end up regurgitating what's been fed to us. TV is full of drama, lying, cheating, stealing, and hurting each other. I avoid watching TV because I don't need to soak up these negative ideas; life is challenging enough without adding to it.

## THINK POSITIVE THOUGHTS

Shedding toxic thoughts from our minds is just as important as decreasing toxic chemicals in and around us for helping us live a Super Life. The fuel for positive thinking comes from focusing on what we want, all the things we are grateful for, and appreciating the lives we live.

Strive to live a long, Super Life filled with positive thoughts, compassionate people, good friends, family, laughter, healthy clean food and water, exercise and fitness, meditation, yoga, sunshine, and love. Avoid situations and people that drag you down and make you feel bad about yourself. Instead, choose to surround yourself with people who support you to be your best self, folks who are proud of who you are, and make you feel good. Consider reaching out to help someone else in need. That act alone will fill you with gratitude for all your blessings. And the more gratitude we have, the happier we feel.

Here's to enjoying a healthy Super Life and having a blast each and every day! Don't worry. Be happy. Be strong. Be amazing.

# METRIC CONVERSIONS

- The recipes in this book have not been tested with metric measurements, so some variations might occur.
- Remember that the weight of dry ingredients varies according to the volume or density factor: 1 cup of flour weighs far less than 1 cup of sugar, and 1 tablespoon doesn't necessarily hold 3 teaspoons.

## — General Formulas for Metric Conversion

| | |
|---|---|
| Ounces to grams | ⇒ ounces × 28.35 = grams |
| Grams to ounces | ⇒ grams × 0.035 = ounces |
| Pounds to grams | ⇒ pounds × 453.5 = grams |
| Pounds to kilograms | ⇒ pounds × 0.45 = kilograms |
| Cups to liters | ⇒ cups × 0.24 = liters |
| Fahrenheit to Celsius | ⇒ (°F − 32) × 5 ÷ 9 = °C |
| Celsius to Fahrenheit | ⇒ (°C × 9) ÷ 5 + 32 = °F |

## — Linear Measurements

½ inch = 1½ cm
1 inch = 2½ cm
6 inches = 15 cm
8 inches = 20 cm
10 inches = 25 cm
12 inches = 30 cm
20 inches = 50 cm

## — Volume (Dry) Measurements

¼ teaspoon = 1 milliliter
½ teaspoon = 2 milliliters
¾ teaspoon = 4 milliliters
1 teaspoon = 5 milliliters
1 tablespoon = 15 milliliters
¼ cup = 59 milliliters
⅓ cup = 79 milliliters
½ cup = 118 milliliters
⅔ cup = 158 milliliters
¾ cup = 177 milliliters
1 cup = 225 milliliters
4 cups or 1 quart = 1 liter
½ gallon = 2 liters
1 gallon = 4 liters

## — Volume (Liquid) Measurements

1 teaspoon = ⅙ fluid ounce = 5 milliliters
1 tablespoon = ½ fluid ounce = 15 milliliters
2 tablespoons = 1 fluid ounce = 30 milliliters
¼ cup = 2 fluid ounces = 60 milliliters
⅓ cup = 2⅔ fluid ounces = 79 milliliters
½ cup = 4 fluid ounces = 118 milliliters
1 cup or ½ pint = 8 fluid ounces = 250 milliliters
2 cups or 1 pint = 16 fluid ounces = 500 milliliters
4 cups or 1 quart = 32 fluid ounces = 1,000 milliliters
1 gallon = 4 liters

## — Oven Temperature Equivalents, Fahrenheit (F) and Celsius (C)

100°F = 38°C
200°F = 95°C
250°F = 120°C
300°F = 150°C
350°F = 180°C
400°F = 205°C
450°F = 230°C

## — Weight (Mass) Measurements

1 ounce = 30 grams
2 ounces = 55 grams
3 ounces = 85 grams
4 ounces = ¼ pound = 125 grams
8 ounces = ½ pound = 240 grams
12 ounces = ¾ pound = 375 grams
16 ounces = 1 pound = 454 grams

# SELECTED REFERENCES

## MCFAS

1. Aoyama, T., Nosaka, N., and Kasai, M. "Research on the nutritional characteristics of medium-chain fatty acids." *J Med Invest.* 2007 Aug; 54(3–4):385–8.

2. Bach, A.C., and Babayan, V.K. "Medium-chain triglycerides: an update." *Am J Clin Nutr.* 1982 Nov; 36(5):950–62.

3. Binnert, C., Pachiaudi, C., Beylot, M., Hans, D., Vandermander, J., Chantre, P., Riou, J.P., and Laville, M. "Influence of human obesity on the metabolic fate of dietary long- and medium-chain triacylglycerols." *Am J Clin Nutr.* 1998 Apr; 67(4):595–601.

4. Dong Y.M., Li, Y., Ning, H., Wang, C., Liu, J.R., and Sun, C.H. [Epub ahead of print]. "High dietary intake of medium-chain fatty acids during pregnancy in rats prevents later-life obesity in their offspring." *J Nutr Biochem.* 2010 Nov 24.

5. Geliebter, A., Torbay, N., Bracco, E.F., Hashim, S.A., and Van Itallie, T.B. "Overfeeding with medium-chain triglyceride diet results in diminished deposition of fat." *Am J Clin Nutr.* 1983 Jan; 37(1):1–4.

6. Han, J., Hamilton, J.A., Kirkland, J.L., Corkey, B.E., and Guo, W. "Medium-chain oil reduces fat mass and down-regulates expression of adipogenic genes in rats." *Obes Res.* 2003 Jun; 11(6):734–44.

7. Moussavi, N., Gavino, V., and Receveur, O. "Could the quality of dietary fat, and not just its quantity, be related to risk of obesity?" *Obesity* (Silver Spring). 2008 Jan; 16(1):7–15.

8. Nagao, K., and Yanagita, T. "Medium-chain fatty acids: functional lipids for the prevention and treatment of the metabolic syndrome." *Pharmacol Res.* 2010 Mar; 61(3):208–12. Epub 2009 Nov 30.

9. Papamandjaris, A.A., MacDougall, D.E., and Jones, P.J. "Medium-chain fatty acid metabolism and energy expenditure: obesity treatment implications." *Life Sci.* 1998; 62(14):1203–15.

10. Scalfi, L., Coltorti A., and Contaldo, F. "Postprandial thermogenesis in lean and obese subjects after meals supplemented with medium-chain and long-chain triglycerides." *Am J Clin Nutr.* 1991 May; 53(5):1130–3.

11. Simón, E., Fernández-Quintela, A., Del Puy Portillo, M., and Del Barrio, A.S. "Effects of medium-chain fatty acids on body composition and protein metabolism in overweight rats." *J Physiol Biochem.* 2000 Dec; 56(4):337–46.

12. St-Onge, M.P., and Jones, P.J. "Physiological effects of medium-chain triglycerides: potential agents in the prevention of obesity." *J Nutr.* 2002 Mar; 132(3):329–32.

13. Takeuchi, H., Sekine, S., Kojima, K., and Aoyama, T. "The application of medium-chain fatty acids: edible oil with a suppressing effect on body fat accumulation." *Asia Pac J Clin Nutr.* 2008; 17 Suppl 1:320–3.

14. Xue, K., Guo, H.W., and Chen, F.L. "Effects of medium-chain fatty acids on weight gain and lipids metabolism in obese rats." *Wei Sheng Yan Jiu.* 2006 Mar; 35(2):187–90.

## PROBIOTICS

1. Blaut, M., and Bischoff, S.C. Epub 2010 Sep 8. Probiotics and obesity. *Ann Nutr Metab.* 2010; 57 Suppl:20–3.

2. Brudnak, M,A. "Weight-loss drugs and supplements: are there safer alternatives?" *Med Hypotheses.* 2002 Jan; 58(1):28–33.

3. Cani, P.D., and Delzenne, N.M. "Gut microflora as a target for energy and metabolic homeostasis." *Curr Opin Clin Nutr Metab Care.* 2007 Nov; 10(6):729–34.

4. ———. "Interplay between obesity and associated metabolic disorders: new insights into the gut microbiota." *Curr Opin Pharmacol.* 2009 Dec; 9(6):737–43. Epub 2009 Jul 21.

5. ———. "The role of the gut microbiota in energy metabolism and metabolic disease." *Curr Pharm Des.* 2009; 15(13):1546–58.

6.  Diamant, M., Blaak, E.E., and de Vos, W.M. [Epub ahead of print]. "Do nutrient-gut-microbiota interactions play a role in human obesity, insulin resistance, and type 2 diabetes?" *Obes Rev*. 2010 Aug 13.

7.  DiBaise, J.K., Zhang, H., Crowell, M.D., Krajmalnik-Brown, R., Decker, G.A., and Rittmann, B.E. "Gut microbiota and its possible relationship with obesity." *Mayo Clin Proc*. 2008 Apr; 83(4):460–9.

8.  Ebringer, L., Ferencík, M., and Krajcovic, J. Epub 2008 Dec 16. "Beneficial health effects of milk and fermented dairy products—review." *Folia Microbiol* (Praha). 2008; 53(5):378–94.

9.  Kadooka, Y., Sato, M., Imaizumi, K., Ogawa, A., Ikuyama, K., Akai, Y., Okano, M., Kagoshima, M., and Tsuchida, T. "Regulation of abdominal adiposity by probiotics (Lactobacillus gasseri SBT2055) in adults with obese tendencies in a randomized controlled trial." *Eur J Clin Nutr*. 2010 Jun; 64(6):636–43. Epub 2010 Mar 10.

10. Kang, J.H., Yun, S.I., and Park, H.O. "Effects of Lactobacillus gasseri BNR17 on body weight and adipose tissue mass in diet-induced overweight rats." *J Microbiol*. 2010 Oct; 48(5):712–4. Epub 2010 Nov 3.

11. Kaur, I.P., Kuhad, A., Garg, A., and Chopra, K. "Probiotics: delineation of prophylactic and therapeutic benefits." *J Med Food*. 2009 Apr; 12(2):219–35.

12. Kondo, S., Xiao, J.Z., Satoh, T., Odamaki, T., Takahashi, S., Sugahara, H., Yaeshima, T., Iwatsuki, K., Kamei, A., and Abe. K. "Anti-obesity effects of Bifidobacterium breve strain B-3 supplementation in a mouse model with high-fat diet-induced obesity." *Biosci Biotechnol Biochem*. 2010; 74(8):1656–61. Epub 2010 Aug 7.

13. Mai, V., and Draganov, P.V. "Recent advances and remaining gaps in our knowledge of associations between gut microbiota and human health." *World J Gastroenterol*. 2009 Jan 7; 15(1):81–5.

14. Musso, G., Gambino, R., and Cassader, M. "Gut microbiota as a regulator of energy homeostasis and ectopic fat deposition: mechanisms and implications for metabolic disorders." *Curr Opin Lipidol*. 2010 Feb; 21(1):76–83.

15. Pataky, Z., Bobbioni-Harsch, E., Hadengue, A., Carpentier, A., and Golay, A. [Gut microbiota, responsible for our body weight?]. [Article in French] *Rev Med Suisse*. 2009 Mar 25; 5(196):662–4, 666.

16. Sanz, Y., Santacruz, A., and De Palma, G. Epub 2008 Dec 3. "Insights into the roles of gut microbes in obesity." *Interdiscip Perspect Infect Dis*. 2008; 2008:829101.

17. Scarpellini, E., Campanale, M., Leone, D., Purchiaroni, F., Vitale, G., Lauritano, E.C., and Gasbarrini, A. "Gut microbiota and obesity." *Intern Emerg Med.* 2010 Oct; 5 Suppl 1:S53–6.

18. Serino, M., Luche, E., Chabo, C., Amar, J., and Burcelin, R. Epub 2009 May 5. "Intestinal microflora and metabolic diseases." *Diabetes Metab.* 2009 Sep; 35(4):262–72.

19. Tennyson, C.A., and Friedman, G. "Microecology, obesity, and probiotics." *Curr Opin Endocrinol Diabetes Obes.* 2008 Oct; 15(5):422–7.

20. Tsai, F., and Coyle, W.J. "The microbiome and obesity: is obesity linked to our gut flora?" *Curr Gastroenterol Rep.* 2009 Aug; 11(4):307–13.

## PREBIOTICS

1. Bengmark, S. "Pre-, pro-, and synbiotics." *Curr Opin Clin Nutr Metab Care.* 2001 Nov; 4(6):571–9.

2. Bengmark, S., and Gil, A. "Bioecological and nutritional control of disease: prebiotics, probiotics and, synbiotics." *Nutr Hosp.* 2006 May; 21 Suppl 2:72–84, 73–86.

3. Cani, P.D., and Delzenne, N.M. "Interplay between obesity and associated metabolic disorders: new insights into the gut microbiota." *Curr Opin Pharmacol.* 2009 Dec; 9(6):737–43. Epub 2009 Jul 21.

4. Cashman, K. "Prebiotics and calcium bioavailability." *Curr Issues Intest Microbiol.* 2003 Mar; 4(1):21–32.

5. "Cholesterol-lowering effects of probiotics and prebiotics: a review of in vivo and in vitro findings." *Int J Mol Sci.* 2010 Jun 17; 11(6):2499–522.

6. Chow, J. "Probiotics and prebiotics: A brief overview." *J Ren Nutr.* 2002 Apr; 12(2):76–86.

7. De Vrese, M. "Health benefits of probiotics and prebiotics in women." *Menopause Int.* 2009 Mar; 15(1):35–40.

8. De Vrese, M., and Schrezenmeir, J. "Probiotics, prebiotics, and synbiotics." *Adv Biochem Eng Biotechnol.* 2008; 111:1–66.

9. Kelly, G. "Inulin-type prebiotics—a review: part 1." *Altern Med Rev.* 2008 Dec; 13 (4):315–29.

10. ———. "Inulin-type prebiotics:—a review: part 2." *Altern Med Rev.* 2009 Mar; 14(1):36–55.

11. Kolida, S., Tuohy, K., and Gibson, G.R. "Prebiotic effects of inulin and oligofructose." *Br J Nutr*. 2002 May; 87 Suppl 2:S193–7.

12. Marti del Moral, A., Moreno-Aliaga, M.J., and Martínez Hernández, J.A. "The effect of prebiotics on lipid metabolism." *Nutr Hosp*. 2003 Jul-Aug; 18(4):181–8.

13. O'Sullivan, L., Murphy, B., McLoughlin, P., Duggan, P., Lawlor, P.G., Hughes, H., and Gardiner, G.E. "Prebiotics from marine macroalgae for human and animal health applications." *Mar Drugs*. 2010 Jul 1; 8(7):2038–64.

14. Pereira, D.I., and Gibson, G.R. "Effects of consumption of probiotics and prebiotics on serum lipid levels in humans." *Crit Rev Biochem Mol Biol*. 2002; 37(4):259–81.

15. Roberfroid, M.B. "Health benefits of nondigestible oligosaccharides." *Adv Exp Med Biol*. 1997; 427:211–9.

16. ———. "Prebiotics and synbiotics: concepts and nutritional properties." *Br J Nutr*. 1998 Oct; 80(4):S197–202.

17. ———. "Prebiotics and probiotics: are they functional foods?" *Am J Clin Nutr*. 2000 Jun; 71(6 Suppl):1682S–7S; discussion 1688S–90S.

18. Roberfroid, M., Gibson, G.R., Hoyles, L., McCartney, A.L., Rastall, R., Rowland, I., Wolvers, D., Watzl, B., Szajewska, H., Stahl, B., Guarner, F., Respondek, F., Whelan, K., Coxam, V., Davicco, M.J., Léotoing, L., Wittrant, Y., Delzenne, N.M., Cani, P.D., Neyrinck, A.M., and Meheust, A. "Prebiotic effects: metabolic and health benefits." *Br J Nutr*. 2010 Aug; 104 Suppl 2:S1–63.

19. Roy, C.C., Kien, C.L., Bouthillier, L., and Levy, E. "Short-chain fatty acids: ready for prime time?" *Nutr Clin Pract*. 2006 Aug; 21(4):351–66.

20. Sabater-Molina, M, Larqué, E., Torrella, F., and Zamora, S. "Dietary fructo-oligosaccharides and potential benefits on health." *J Physiol Biochem*. 2009 Sep; 65(3):315–28.

21. Schley, P.D., and Field, C.J. "The immune-enhancing effects of dietary fibres and prebiotics." *Br J Nutr*. 2002 May; 87 Suppl 2:S221–30.

22. Simmering, R. and Blaut, M. "Pro- and prebiotics—the tasty guardian angels?" *Appl Microbiol Biotechnol*. 2001 Jan; 55(1):19–28.

23. Wong, J.M., de Souza, R., Kendall, C.W., Emam, A., and Jenkins, D.J. "Colonic health: fermentation and short-chain fatty acids." *J Clin Gastroenterol*. 2006 Mar; 40(3):235–43.

24. Zinn, A.R. "Unconventional wisdom about the obesity epidemic." *Am J Med Sci*. 2010 Dec; 340 (6):481–91.

## RAW AND PLANT-BASED DIETS

1. Aslam, M.N., Bhagavathula, N., Paruchuri, T., et al. "Growth-inhibitory effects of a mineralized extract from the red marine algae, Lithothamnion calcareum, on Ca2+-sensitive and Ca2+-resistant human colon carcinoma cells." *Cancer Lett*. 2009 October 8; 283(2):186–92.

2. Cumashi, A., Ushakova, N.A., Preobrazhenskaya, M.E., et al. "A comparative study of the anti-inflammatory, anticoagulant, antiangiogenic, and antiadhesive activities of nine different fucoidans from brown seaweeds." *Glycobiology*. 2007; 17(5):541–52.

3. Cunningham, E. "What is a raw foods diet and are there any risks or benefits associated with it?" *J Am Diet Assoc*. 2004 Oct; 104(10):1623.

4. de Vos, R.H., and Blijleven, W.G. "The effect of processing conditions on glucosinolates in cruciferous vegetables." *Z Lebensm Unters Forsch*. 1988 Dec; 187(6):525–9.

5. Elvevoll, E.O., and Osterud, B. "Impact of processing on nutritional quality of marine food items." *Forum Nutr*. 2003; 56:337–40.

6. Ganesh, E.A., Das, S., Arun, G. et al. "Heparin-like compound from green algae Chaetomorpha antennina—as potential anticoagulant agent." *Asian J Med Sci*. 2009; 1(3):114–6.

7. Hobbs, S.H. "Attitudes, practices, and beliefs of individuals consuming a raw foods diet." *Explore* (NY). 2005 Jul; 1(4):272–7.

8. Martinez-Villaluenga, C., Peñas, E., Frias, J., Ciska, E., Honke, J., Piskula, M.K., Kozlowska, H., and Vidal-Valverde, C. "Influence of fermentation conditions on glucosinolates, ascorbigen, and ascorbic acid content in white cabbage (Brassica oleracea var. capitata cv. Taler) cultivated in different seasons." *J Food Sci*. 2009 Jan-Feb; 74(1):C62–7.

9. Nus, M., Ruperto, M., and Sánchez-Muniz, F.J. [Nuts, cardio, and cerebrovascular risks. A Spanish perspective]. *Arch Latinoam Nutr*. 2004 Jun; 54(2):137–48.

10. Payne, M.J., Hurst, W.J., Miller, K.B., Rank, C., and Stuart, D.A. "Impact of fermentation, drying, roasting, and Dutch processing on epicatechin and catechin content of cacao beans and cocoa ingredients." *J Agric Food Chem*. 2010 Oct 13; 58(19):10518–27.

11. Potter, J.D., and Steinmetz, K. "Vegetables, fruit, and phytoestrogens as preventive agents." *IARC Sci Publ*. 1996; 139:61–90.

12. Satia, J.A., Kristal, A.R., Patterson, R.E., Neuhouser, M.L., and Trudeau, E. "Psychosocial factors and dietary habits associated with vegetable consumption." *Nutrition*. 2002 Mar; 18(3):247–54.

13. Vadlapudi, V., and Naidu, K.C. "In vitro bioevaluation of antioxidant activities of selected marine algae." *J Pharm Res*. 2010; 3(2):329–331.

14. Xu, J.G., Hu, Q.P., Duan, J.L., and Tian, C.R. "Dynamic changes in gamma-aminobutyric acid and glutamate decarboxylase activity in oats (Avena nuda L.) during steeping and germination." *J Agric Food Chem*. 2010 Sep 8; 58(17):9759–63.

15. Young-Joo, L., Adlercreutz, H., and Kwon, H.J. "Quantitative analysis of isoflavones and lignans in sea vegetables consumed in Korea using isotope dilution gas chromatography-mass spectrometry." *Food Sci Biotech*. 2006; 15(1):102–6

## THERMOGENESIS

1. Carson, T. "What are the health benefits of Capsaicin?" Last updated 2011 June 20. www.livestrong.com/article/342597.

2. Chan She Ping-Delfos, W., and Soares, M. "Diet-induced thermogenesis, fat oxidation, and food intake following sequential meals: influence of calcium and vitamin D." *Clin Nutr*. 2011 Jun; 30(3):376–83. Epub 2011 Jan 26.

3. Gruenwald, J., Freder, J., and Armbruester, N. "Cinnamon and Health." *Crit Rev Food Sci Nutr*. 2010 Oct; 50(9):822–34.

4. Lee, M.S., Kim, I.H., Kim, C.T., and Kim, Y. "Reduction of body weight by dietary garlic is associated with an increase of uncoupling protein mRNA expression and activation of AMP-activated protein kinase in diet-induced obese mice." *J Nutr*. 2011 Sep 14. [Epub ahead of print].

5. Matsui, N., Ito, R., Nishimura, E., Yoshikawa, M., Kato, M., Kamei, M., Shibata, H., Matsumoto, I., Abe, K., and Hashizume, S. "Ingested cocoa can prevent high-fat diet-induced obesity by regulating the expression of genes for fatty acid metabolism." *Nutrition*. 2005 May; 21(5):594–601.

6. Medvedik, S. "Thermogenic Foods List." 2011 March 28. www.livestrong.com/article/198798.

7. Murase, T., Haramizu, S., Shimotoyodome, A., Nagasawa, A., and Tokimitsu, I. "Green tea extract improves endurance capacity and increases muscle lipid

oxidation in mice." *Am J Physiol Regul Integr Comp Physiol.* 2004 Nov 24. [Epub ahead of print].

8. Nagao, T., Komine, Y., Soga, S., Meguro, S., Hase, T., Tanaka, Y., and Tokimitsu, I. "Ingestion of a tea rich in catechins leads to a reduction in body fat and malondialdehyde-modified LDL in men." *Am J Clin Nutr.* 2005 Jan; 81(1):122–9.

9. Shixian, Q., VanCrey, B., Shi, J., Kakuda, Y., and Jiang, Y. "Green tea extract thermogenesis-induced weight loss by epigallocatechin gallate inhibition of catechol-O-methyltransferase." *J Med Food.* 2006 Winter; 9(4):451–8.

10. Westerterp-Plantenga, M.S. "The significance of protein in food intake and body weight regulation." *Curr Opin Clin Nutr Metab Care.* 2003 Nov; 6(6):635–8.

# ACKNOWLEDGMENTS

Thank you to my mother Meejung Jae Phyo and my late father Inchol Joseph Phyo for teaching me early on that our health is our most valuable asset, and that money can't buy health, wellness, happiness, or longevity. My brother Max, thank you for being my biggest supporter and for taking part in Mom's testing group with me, tasting the most potent, sometimes not-so-delicious, vegetable juices and good-for-us treats that have given us our vitality today.

Heather Jackson, thank you for believing in me and my vision, for being my sounding board, for helping me organize my thoughts, and for getting all my ducks lined up neatly in a row. It was a huge honor and pleasure to work with you. Thank you to my team and family at DaCapo: Renee Sedliar, Kate Burke, Lindsey Triebel, Kevin Hanover, Alex Camlin, and Mark Corsey. Love working with you all. Thank you Shadi Azarpour and Eric Weissler for your unwavering support and love, for always standing by my side. Shadi, you are a blessing to me. Thank you to my ICM agents Tina Wexler and Andrea Barzvi.

To my crew of SmartMonkey® recipe testers and to everyone who participated in my test groups, thank you, especially John Johnson, Jennifer M. S. Robertson, and Siel Ju. Thank you Diane Paylor for all your love, support, for believing in me, and for being part of my family.

Antonio Sanchez, thank you for your amazing illustrations that grace all of my books. You're the best illustrator in the world. Thank you to all my friends and experts who contributed inspiration and recipes, including Robert Cheeke, Philip McCluskey, Penni Shelton, Angela Stokes-Monarch, and Tonya Zavasta.

A special thank you to Dr. Richard DeAndrea and John Wood for teaching me long ago about the power of raw foods for detoxing and cleansing, with the side effect of weight loss, and for showing me how to heal myself and others with food as medicine.

As always, thank you Kanga, my dog, for reminding me to stop to smell the flowers, to bask in the sunlight, to play, and to nap.

Thank you, the reader, for picking up this book and having confidence that its contents will help to make you healthier and happier. May you achieve your ideal weight, feel amazing, look radiant, feel blissful, and live a long Super Life!

# 15-Day Menu Plan

| DAY | Breakfast | Snack | Lunch |
|---|---|---|---|
| 1 | Blueberry Blast | Pineapple Green Shake | Spicy Bok Choy Soup |
| 2 | Simple Strawberry Shake | Apple Green Mar-tea-ni | Ginger Soup |
| 3 | Pina Colada | Pear Power Shake | Spicy Avocado Soup |
| 4 | Ginger Mango Shake | Ginger Mango Shake (drink) or Grapefruit Salad (eat) | Easy Being Green Salad |
| 5 | Banana Shake | Banana Shake or Pomegranate Blueberry Salad | Spring Sauerkraut Salad with Thermo Dressing |
| 6 | Chocolate Banana Mylk Shake | Chocolate Banana Mylk Shake or Pineapple Coconut Salad | Asian Cabbage Salad with Apple Cider Vinaigrette |
| 7 | Matcha Shake | Matcha Shake or Pecan Candy Apple | Corn and Basil Mesclun Salad with Thermo Dressing or Apple Cider Vinaigrette |
| 8 | Vanilla Blueberry Shake | Vanilla Blueberry Shake or Red, White, and Blue Berry Salad | Kreamy Chipotle Salad with Kreamy Chipotle Dressing |
| 9 | Pineapple Cilantro Shake | Pineapple Cilantro Shake or Cucumber Guacamole | Cabbage Salad with Cucumber Miso Dressing |
| 10 | Pear Lime Ginger Shake | Pear Lime Ginger Shake or Watermelon Grapefruit Salad | Zucchini Hummus |
| 11 | Green Grapefruit Shake | Green Grapefruit Shake or Mint and Basil Tropical Fruit Salad | Shredded Sesame Salad with Orange Ginger Vinaigrette |
| 12 | Orange Vanilla Shake | Orange Vanilla Shake or Peach Crumble | Italian Salad |
| 13 | Avocado Shake | Avocado Shake or Fudge Brownie with Fresh Berries | Fennel Slaw with Dill Vinaigrette |
| 14 | Beauty Berry Shake | Beauty Berry Shake or Trail Mix Cookies | Cumin Slaw with Coconut Miso Vinaigrette |
| 15 | Choose shake | Choose shake or snack | Choose salad |

| Snack | Dinner | Snack |
|-------|--------|-------|
| Shake or soup | Tomato Bisque | Leftover soup |
| Shake or soup | Marvelous Minestrone | Leftover soup |
| Shake or soup | Curry Coconut Soup | Leftover soup |
| Strawberry Mint Shake | Red Pepper Soup | Soup, ½ avocado, or nuts |
| Pineapple Protein Shake | Kreamy Dill Delight | Soup, ½ avocado, or nuts |
| Mango Mint Shake | Coconut Tomato Soup | Soup, ½ avocado, or nuts |
| Smooth Operator | Souper Supper | Soup, ½ avocado, or nuts |
| Kreamy Cucumber Soup or Vanilla Blueberry Shake | Zucchini Noodles with Marinara Sauce | Soup, ½ avocado, or nuts |
| Garlic Bell Soup or Pineapple Cilantro Shake | Celery Almond Paté | Soup, ½ avocado, or nuts |
| Curried Cilantro Cucumber Soup or Pear Lime Ginger Shake | Mixed Vegetable Seaweed Rolls with Sesame Dipping Sauce | Soup, ½ avocado, or nuts |
| Coconut Miso Soup or Green Grapefruit Shake | Collard Rolls with Cashew Paté | Soup, ½ avocado, or nuts |
| Curried Zucchini Cucumber Soup or Orange Vanilla Shake | Marinated Mushrooms in Lettuce Wraps | Soup, ½ avocado, or nuts |
| Carrot Ginger Soup or Avocado Shake | Pesto Wraps | Soup, ½ avocado, or nuts |
| Kreamy Tomato Gazpacho or Beauty Berry Shake | Mushroom Rolls with Root Rice | Soup, ½ avocado, or nuts |
| Choose soup or shake | Choose soup or dinner meal | Soup, ½ avocado, or nuts |

*What challenged you today?*

------------------------------------

------------------------------------

------------------------------------

------------------------------------

------------------------------------

*How do you feel?*

------------------------------------

------------------------------------

------------------------------------

------------------------------------

------------------------------------

------------------------------------

------------------------------------

------------------------------------

------------------------------------

------------------------------------

------------------------------------

------------------------------------

------------------------------------

*What challenged you today?*

....................................................................................................

....................................................................................................

....................................................................................................

....................................................................................................

....................................................................................................

*How do you feel?*

....................................................................................................

....................................................................................................

....................................................................................................

....................................................................................................

....................................................................................................

....................................................................................................

....................................................................................................

....................................................................................................

....................................................................................................

....................................................................................................

....................................................................................................

....................................................................................................

....................................................................................................

....................................................................................................

....................................................................................................

## What challenged you today?

......................................................................

......................................................................

......................................................................

......................................................................

......................................................................

## How do you feel?

......................................................................

......................................................................

......................................................................

......................................................................

......................................................................

......................................................................

......................................................................

......................................................................

......................................................................

......................................................................

......................................................................

......................................................................

......................................................................

......................................................................

# INDEX

# RECIPE INDEX